REGULATING ALCOHOL AROUND THE WORLD

D1711088

Solving Social Problems

Series Editor:
Bonnie Berry, Director of the Social Problems Research Group, USA

Solving Social Problems provides a forum for the description and measurement of social problems, with a keen focus on the concrete remedies proposed for their solution. The series takes an international perspective, exploring social problems in various parts of the world, with the central concern being always their possible remedy. As such, work is welcomed on subjects as diverse as environmental damage, terrorism, economic disparities and economic devastation, poverty, inequalities, domestic assaults and sexual abuse, health care, natural disasters, labour inequality, animal abuse, crime, and mental illness and its treatment. In addition to recommending solutions to social problems, the books in this series are theoretically sophisticated, exploring previous discussions of the issues in question, examining other attempts to resolve them, and adopting and discussing methodologies that are commonly used to measure social problems. Proposed solutions may be framed as changes in policy, practice, or more broadly, social change and social movement. Solutions may be reflective of ideology, but are always pragmatic and detailed, explaining the means by which the suggested solutions might be achieved.

Also in the series

The Evidence Enigma
Correctional Boot Camps and Other Failures in Evidence-Based Policymaking
Tiffany Bergin

Street Practice
Changing the Lens on Poverty and Public Assistance
Lori McNeil

Prison Violence
Causes, Consequences and Solutions
Kristine Levan

Borderline Slavery
Mexico, United States, and the Human Trade
Edited by Susan Tiano and Moira Murphy-Aguilar with Brianne Bigej

Regulating Alcohol around the World

Policy Cocktails

TIFFANY BERGIN
Kent State University, USA

ASHGATE

Published by
Ashgate Publishing Limited
Wey Court East
Union Road
Farnham
Surrey, GU9 7PT
England

Ashgate Publishing Company
110 Cherry Street
Suite 3-1
Burlington, VT 05401-3818
USA

www.ashgate.com

British Library Cataloguing in Publication Data
A catalogue record for this book is available from the British Library

The Library of Congress has cataloged the printed edition as follows:
Bergin, Tiffany.
  Regulating alcohol around the world : policy cocktails / by Tiffany Bergin.
     pages cm. -- (Solving social problems)
  Includes bibliographical references.
  ISBN 978-1-4094-4525-8 (hardback) -- ISBN 978-1-4094-4526-5 (ebook) -- ISBN 978-1-4724-0262-2 (epub) 1. Drinking of alcoholic beverages--Government policy--History. 2. Alcoholism--Social aspects. 3. Controlled drinking. 4. Temperance. I. Title.
  HV5081.B47 2013
  363.4'1--dc23

                                                                              2013002710

ISBN 9781409445258 (hbk)
ISBN 9781409445265 (ebk – PDF)
ISBN 9781472402622 (ebk – ePUB)

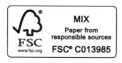

Printed in the United Kingdom by Henry Ling Limited, at the Dorset Press, Dorchester, DT1 1HD

Contents

Acknowledgments   *vii*

1   Introduction   1

2   Research into Alcohol's Social Harms   13

3   Alcohol and Policymaking   27

4   History, Culture, Context, and Transformation   43

5   Key Lessons from Prohibition Policies: Beyond the 1920s   57

6   General Efforts to Reduce Alcohol's Social Harms   71

7   Targeted Policies: Minimum Drinking Age Laws   85

8   Concluding Thoughts   103

Bibliography   *111*
Index   *153*

This book is dedicated to Tita Bautista and Kate Bergin

Acknowledgments

I am very grateful to Chris McConnell whose advice and assistance greatly improved this work. I am also thankful for the suggestions of Bonnie Berry, the editor of the *Solving Social Problems* book series, as well as Neil Jordan and Kayleigh Huelin at Ashgate. Some of the research contained in this book was completed while I was Sutasoma Trust Research Fellow at Lucy Cavendish College, University of Cambridge. I am very grateful to both the Trust and the College for their support. As always, I am thankful for the unwavering guidance and support of Pamela Huttenberg and Brent D. Bergin. Of course, as author, the contents of this book are my responsibility alone.

Chapter 1

Introduction

In late April 2012, a commentator argued in *The Malaysian Insider* that "Alcohol consumption will not stop, and what policymakers must concentrate on is changing the environment so persons who consume alcohol do not drink excessively, and that they are protected from alcohol-related harm" (Rahman, 2012).

Just over a week later, a Canadian newspaper article reported Quebec's decision to join Ontario in imposing a blood-alcohol limit of zero for young drivers (Aylward, 2012). In the article, an activist said of the policy: "Places like Ontario have seen a significant drop in deaths and injuries right across the board, including young drivers. It's working."

That same day, Brazil's Senate approved legislation allowing alcohol to be sold in stadiums during the 2014 World Cup—even though alcohol sales at matches have been banned since 2003 ("Brazil Senate ...", 2012). The passage of the legislation was controversial, with one Brazilian senator declaring that even though he voted for the bill he felt "violence in stadiums has decreased a lot because of the ban against alcoholic beverages."

Six days later, a commentator in the British newspaper *The Guardian* questioned Scotland's decision to impose a minimum unit price for alcoholic beverages, writing: "Will minimum pricing make us drink less? It is very unlikely that minimum pricing will affect David Cameron's chaotic problem drinkers; some problems need deep solutions and some are not solvable at all" (Gold, 2012).

Two days after that, Kenya's Presidential Cabinet voted in favor of tougher penalties for driving under the influence of alcohol among other driving offenses, with the goal of reducing fatal traffic accidents in that country (Ohito, 2012).

Less than a week later, an Australian politician stated that he and other members of a parliamentary committee had "received evidence that alcohol labels need to be introduced as part of a wider health promotion strategy and also evidence that alcohol labels don't work," prior to a series of governmental discussions on the issue (as quoted in "Alcohol warnings ...", 2012).

These six examples—from six continents during a single four-week period— illustrate the centrality of alcohol-related policymaking in twenty-first century society. The harm reduction strategies, blood-alcohol limits for drivers, retail bans, minimum prices, tougher penalties, and warning labels for alcoholic beverages discussed in these examples are just six of the myriad kinds of alcohol policies that policymakers, practitioners, activists, commentators, and citizens around the world debate on a regular basis. These debates often revolve around questions of evidence and effectiveness, as the examples above illustrate. Which policies are most effective at reducing alcohol's social harms? What evidence is there of a particular policy's success? Yet evidence is not the only force that can impact alcohol policymaking. History and culture can matter as well, as can political and economic forces such as globalization. Exploring the impacts of all of these factors on alcohol policymaking across time and around the world is this book's central task.

Alcohol is a global concern, and policy decisions about alcohol are made in an increasingly-globalized context. Recognizing this—and warning that alcohol contributes to at least 2.5 million global deaths per year—the World Health Organization (WHO) in 2010 unveiled its Global Strategy to target harmful alcohol consumption. The strategy aims to increase awareness of alcohol's harms and to promote the implementation of practices that can most effectively tackle these harms (p. 8). Such policies include establishing price incentives for non-alcoholic drinks, regulating the hours during which retail sales of alcohol can take place, and enacting minimum age limits for purchase (pp. 9–23). At the moment, however, these policies are only recommendations and no country is required to adopt them (Sridhar, 2012).

The WHO has long emphasized an international approach to tackling alcohol's social harms. Twenty-seven years before the release of the Global Strategy, in 1983, the WHO's decision-making body pronounced alcohol one of the world's foremost health hazards (Jernigan et al., 2000, p. 491). The WHO's approach is also based on rigorous empirical research. Indeed, in the years leading up to the adoption of the Global Strategy, the organization's Secretariat released a report entitled *Evidence-Based Strategies and Interventions to Reduce Alcohol-Related Harm* (WHO, 2007). An evidence-based approach is also endorsed by other supra-national bodies. In its 2006 alcohol strategy, the European Commission advised EU member states that, when it comes to measures to control alcohol misuse, "every measure has to be considered on a case-by-case basis; in all cases, they should be evidence-based" (p. 14). The United Nations' Office on Drugs and Crime has undertaken reviews and disseminated lists of "evidence-based" programs to prevent the misuse of alcohol and other drugs (2009, p. 2).

National governments have also promoted the importance of evidence-based policies and practices to reduce alcohol's social harms. As early as the 1980s, the Dutch government emphasized an evidence-based approach to combat the harmful use of alcohol (Bongers, 1998, p. 44). In more recent years, Ireland's Health Service Executive issued the report *Towards a Framework for Implementing Evidence Based Alcohol Interventions* (Barry and Armstrong, 2011), while Hong Kong's Department of Health *Action Plan to Reduce Alcohol-Related Harm* is said to be "built on detailed examination of the local situation on alcohol use, while drawing references from overseas *evidence* as well as recommendations of the WHO" (2011, p. v; emphasis added). A recent announcement on the Scottish government's (2012) website proclaimed that the "Scottish Government is developing interventions which are informed by a strong evidence base." Meanwhile, Bermuda's Department for National Drug Control has underlined the importance of implementing "evidence-based substance abuse services throughout the criminal justice system" to tackle dependencies on alcohol or other drugs.

As these examples illustrate, many governments have, unsurprisingly, expressed interest in evidence-based strategies to combat alcohol's social harms. Such interest ostensibly matches the recommendations of numerous researchers from around the world who have argued that "policies should be based on scientific evidence showing the effectiveness of various alcohol policy options" (König and Segura, 2011, p. 49). However, endorsing evidence-based rhetoric is one thing—actually adopting and implementing evidence-based practices is quite another. What political, economic, historical, cultural, and other factors impede the adoption and implementation of evidence-based alcohol strategies? Do theories from other policymaking literatures offer insight into the forces that influence alcohol policies? What lessons can countries learn from past experiences?

Building on the small but growing literature on alcohol policymaking, this book explores historical and contemporary case studies to gain a richer understanding of the factors that impact alcohol policies around the world. The explanatory value of leading theories from political science, policy studies, and other fields is assessed, and research about the cross-national transfer of policies and beliefs about evidence is presented. The book therefore adopts a global, historical, and interdisciplinary perspective to examine the critical issue of alcohol policymaking. Despite the issue's prominence in contemporary societal debates, and despite landmark related work by Stevens (2007), Schrad (2010), Room (1991), Johnson and colleagues (2004), and other scholars, the alcohol policymaking process still strongly needs more attention from researchers. This book therefore offers researchers, practitioners, students, and other stakeholders, a highly accessible synthesis of existing works and studies, illuminating the many forces that shape alcohol policy decisions. The book also advances guidance for policymakers about how evidence can best inform policymaking, as well as summarizing lessons that can be learned from previous efforts to change alcohol policies.

Key Themes

Policies that address alcohol's *social harms* are the focus of this volume. Room's (2000, p. 94) definition of *social harm* as a "perceived misperformance or failure to perform in major social roles—as a family member, as a worker, as a friend or neighbour, or in terms of public demeanour" is employed here. This broad definition is used to capture the range of negative consequences that can result from alcohol misuse. In particular, long-term health impacts to drinkers, violence, traffic accidents, and other impacts are explored in detail.

The severity of these various kinds of harms underlines the importance of the research discussed in this book. Alcohol consumption has been found to play a causal role in at least 60 different medical conditions (Room et al., 2005), and the WHO reports that four percent of global deaths are due to alcohol (2011b, p. 20).

Alcohol may be involved in nearly a third of homicide deaths and a quarter of suicides (Smith et al., 1999) and one report based upon US data found that alcohol was involved in almost 40 percent of violent victimizations (Greenfeld, 1998). Alcohol may increase the incidence and severity of domestic violence (Leonard and Quigley, 1999; Testa et al., 2003) and produce serious developmental and cognitive deficits following excessive prenatal exposure (Fast and Conry, 2009).

Researchers have long studied these social harms. Indeed, the American physician Benjamin Rush, Surgeon General in George Washington's army and a close friend of John and Abigail Adams, pioneered the idea of "addiction" to alcohol in the 1780s and 1790s (Butterfield, 1950; Ferentzy, 2001). One of his works from this period, *An Inquiry into the Effects of Spirituous Liquors on the Human Body* (1785), was among the earliest comprehensive attempts to "medicalize" the study of alcohol abuse. In this publication Rush described the relative dangers of different types of alcoholic beverages and connected excessive alcohol consumption to pneumonia, tuberculosis, and other medical conditions; some of these links have since been proven by contemporary studies (Lönnroth et al., 2008; Rehm et al., 2009; Szabo et al., 1997).

Although research about alcohol policymaking is still nascent, research into alcohol's social harms has a long history, and enthusiasm for *applying* this research to policy has increased in recent decades in many parts of the world. As Babor (2002) has reported, cross-national collaboration in alcohol research—often conducted under the auspices of major public health bodies such as the WHO—has grown dramatically since the 1970s; such research has helped foster a new "what works" culture that is focused on identifying and applying effective policies and programs to reduce alcohol's social harms.

Of course not all of alcohol's potential social harms can be addressed in one volume. Instead, this book presents case studies of attempts to: sharply reduce (and even prohibit) the sale of alcohol; reduce alcohol's social harms *in general* without prohibiting alcohol; target specific social harms related to alcohol misuse; and address multiple specific social harms in concert. The details of each case study are first explored. Then theories from the general policymaking literature and various research traditions are applied to each case to test their explanatory value. Finally, wider lessons are then identified from the case studies, including lessons about how to better facilitate the inclusion of research evidence in policy decisions. To show how such ideas are explored in this book, the next section presents an introductory case study. This case study illustrates the contemporary challenges of alcohol policymaking, and highlights several essential themes that are revisited in future chapters.

A Case Study: Pine Ridge and Whiteclay

Approximately 4.5 million cans of beer are sold each year in Whiteclay, Nebraska—a town with a population of just 14 people (Melecki, 2009). Demand for alcohol is so high in the town that a *New York Times* reporter recently noted that beer prices there were higher than in New York City (Williams, 2012). Whiteclay's location is the reason for these anomalies. The town lies close to Nebraska's border with South Dakota; on the other side of that border is the Pine Ridge Reservation, which was established in the late nineteenth century, belongs to the Oglala Sioux Nation, and is the second-largest Native American reservation in the US (Oglala Sioux Tribe, 2012). Nearly half of the reservation's population lives below the poverty line (Ford, 2011). Some 80 percent of adults are unemployed (Oglala Sioux Tribe Department of Public Safety, 2010). Only 10 percent of young people finish high school and tuberculosis rates are around eight times higher than the US average (Kristof, 2012b). The average life expectancy on the reservation is between just 45 and 52 years—lower than in Haiti and Iraq (Gadkari, 2012; WHO, 2012a, 2012b).

Alcohol's social harms are particularly evident at Pine Ridge, where fetal alcohol spectrum disorders affect a quarter of children born on the reservation, and tribal law enforcement made 20,000 alcohol-related arrests in 2011—even though Pine Ride has a population of just 45,000 (Williams, 2012). Dealing with alcohol-related offences further burdens the already-stretched resources of the Oglala Sioux Tribe Department of Public Safety (2010); the Department is so busy that its officers do not have partners—they must make patrols on their own.

The prevalence of alcohol-related social harms in Pine Ridge is even more striking because alcohol is officially banned on the reservation's grounds. In 1832, the US federal government prohibited Native Americans from consuming alcohol outside of reservations; more than a century later, in 1953, the federal government overturned this ban and also, for the first time, effectively gave tribes authority to regulate alcohol policies on their reservations (May, 1977). Yet the Oglala Sioux initially maintained a ban on alcohol possession and sale at Pine Ridge, before briefly legalizing alcohol in 1969; however, a year later legalization was repealed, and ever since then prohibition has existed within the reservation's grounds (May, 1977, p. 221).

Although the Oglala Sioux have achieved some success in reducing alcohol dependence through prevention and rehabilitation programs emphasizing traditional Sioux spiritual practices and cultural values (Kristof, 2012b), the abundance of alcohol sales in the nearby town of Whiteclay has complicated efforts to enforce prohibition at Pine Ridge. In the 1990s, the unsolved murders of several tribe members in Whiteclay underlined the troubled links between the two communities (Gadkari, 2012). Further conflict can be seen in the 1999 arrests of nine people who were protesting the unsolved murders and alcohol sales, and in the 2007 arrests of three people who were trying to blockade the border between South Dakota and Nebraska (Montag, 2012).

Increasingly frustrated, in February 2012 the tribe initiated a lawsuit in US federal court, seeking $500 million compensation from the multinational alcohol producer Anheuser-Busch and a number of other brewers, as well as several alcohol retail outlets in Whiteclay; the defendants were accused of facilitating the illegal sale and transport of alcohol to the reservation (Williams, 2012). The tribe's objectives in bringing the lawsuit included securing compensation for the costs of treating alcohol-related diseases and medical issues, as well as the costs of deploying law enforcement to deal with alcohol-related crime. Additionally, the tribe has also sought to impose restrictions on alcohol sales in Whiteclay, making it more difficult for tribe members to purchase alcohol there and transport it to the reservation (Wirthman, 2012).

In response to the lawsuit, a lawyer representing one of the defendants—an alcohol retailer in Whiteclay—argued that, if the lawsuit were successful, the retailers would have to "refuse the sale of their otherwise publicly available goods to members of the Oglala Sioux Tribe who live on the Pine Ridge Indian Reservation based solely on their race and ethnicity" (as quoted in Schulte, 2012). A different lawyer for another alcohol retailer in Whiteclay asserted that the stores could not be responsible for alcohol's social harms in Pine Ridge when so many other people were involved in the purchase, transfer, resale, and consumption of alcohol at the reservation (Schulte, 2012). At the time of writing, the lawsuit has yet to be resolved.

This case study highlights several themes that are central to contemporary alcohol policymaking. The first theme is *corporate responsibility*. To what extent are brewers and alcohol retailers—such as those involved in the trade in Whiteclay—responsible for alcohol's social harms? The lawyer for one alcohol retailer in Whiteclay asserted that a court victory for the tribe would mean that manufacturers of alcohol "would be forced to analyze the sales data of each and every one of its distributors and retailers to ensure that it was not selling too much of a product such that it was exposing itself to possible liability for public nuisance"—perhaps an impossible feat (as quoted in Schulte, 2012). On the other side, however, a professor of business ethics asserted that "the liquor stores in this case make money by selling alcohol to a community that has a very serious problem with alcoholism and everything that goes with it … When companies are not paying the full social costs of their activities, they have a special responsibility to mitigate the damage that they do" (Hussain, 2012). This debate about the responsibilities and influence of the alcohol industry is revisited later in this book.

The second related issue raised by this case is that of both the principle and practicalities of *regulation* in a capitalist market. Proponents of neoliberal capitalism are traditionally resistant to many kinds of market regulations, and the questions of whether it would be fair and consistent with the values of a market economy to more rigorously regulate alcohol sales in Whiteclay have prompted much debate. Many commentators have questioned whether such regulations would even be workable. For example, a business school professor observed in a *New York Times* debate about the case: "It is difficult to hold the beer companies responsible for selling a legal product. Even if they wanted to be 'socially responsible,' it's hard for them to avoid selling beer to these consumers near dry reservations, or to smugglers" (Karnani, 2012). Another commentator doubted whether Pine Ridge Reservation's strategy of complete alcohol prohibition was workable at all, and noted that even if alcohol outlets in Whiteclay closed, individuals from Pine Ridge would just drive "farther to another town to purchase beer, increasing the risk of drinking and driving" (Newman, 2012). These statements highlight the difficulties communities face when trying to implement their own alcohol regulations, for even though Pine Ridge instituted prohibition, the availability of alcoholic beverages in nearby Whiteclay undermined this ban. More generally, increased emphasis on free trade around the world and better transportation have complicated communities'— and even whole countries'—efforts to maintain their own alcohol regulations. Increasingly globalization has made it ever-more difficult for countries to restrict cross-border trade in alcoholic beverages. The impact of these free-trade pressures on alcohol polices is examined in detail in Chapter 6.

Of course, the case of Pine Ridge and Whiteclay also raises a third issue: the important role that *history* can play in contemporary alcohol controversies. The Oglala Sioux have a proud but also painful history. The ghost dances of Oglala Sioux and the tribe's 1876 victory at the Battle of Little Bighorn are legendary; however, the infamous Wounded Knee Massacre also took place at Pine Ridge in 1890 (Wirthman, 2012). Given this history and the racism that the Oglala Sioux have faced, it is not surprising that the current case has prompted strong reactions, and perhaps can even be seen as the latest round in an ongoing culture clash between two societies. A member of the Winnebago Tribe (located in Nebraska), for example, wrote that the "free enterprise mumbo jumbo spewed by public officials serves no purpose other than to reassure good ol' boys and the liquor industry that all is O.K. as long as the victims of murder, rape and exploitation at Whiteclay are not white" (LaMere, 2012). The *New York Times* columnist Nicholas Kristof (2012a) pointedly wrote: "After seeing Anheuser-Busch's devastating exploitation of American Indians, I'm done with its beer. The human toll is evident here in Whiteclay." For many readers of his column, Kristof's use of the word "exploitation" may have prompted allusions to the broader history of exploitation of Native Americans by the US government and non-indigenous groups. Kristof's statement therefore illustrates the underlying connections that sometimes exist between contemporary alcohol issues and larger historical forces. The importance of historical context in understanding alcohol policy debates is a theme that is revisited later in this book.

Although Kristof's proposed boycott of Anheuser-Busch received some media attention (Yudell, 2012), not every reaction to his articles was entirely positive, further underlining the complexities of the issues in this area. For example, the founder of the Native American Journalists Association wrote that "Nick Kristof's heart was in the right place, but he didn't look far enough" to seek out views from tribal leaders and key figures in the numerous community groups and institutions on the reservation that are working hard to overcome poverty, alcohol misuse, and other societal challenges (Giago, 2012). The importance of recognizing these efforts was emphasized by one member of the tribe, whose children had recently graduated from high school, and who told a reporter from the *Denver Post*: "I am Oglala Lakota. I am neither a statistic to be put on a chart, nor are my children … We see the stats, we know them, we are related to them, we live them, we are them.

But we are also the ones who must save ourselves" (as quoted in Wirthman, 2012). Human societies are, of course, incredibly multifaceted and it is essential to remember that generalizations about drinking patterns or alcohol's social harms are just that—generalizations that can mask interesting nuances. Such nuances equally deserve attention from researchers.

The fourth and final theme related to the case that needs to be reviewed here is how the *inherited wisdom or perceived lessons of history* can affect how alcohol issues are framed in policy. The most dramatic alcohol policy change in American history took place in 1919 when the Volstead Act was passed and the Eighteenth Amendment was ratified, thereby outlawing the manufacture and sale of alcohol in the US beginning the following year; however, just 13 years after it came into force, the Eighteenth Amendment was repealed, bringing an end to the Prohibition Era (Hamm, 1995). Today, Prohibition—associated with gangsters and speakeasies—is largely viewed as a failure. As Schrad (2010, p. 3) has emphatically put it: "The prohibition of alcohol was a mistake—a historic policy gaffe and a political fiasco." Prohibition's perceived failures continue to cast a shadow over many contemporary American debates about alcohol policymaking. "It has been seventy-five years since the Prohibition era," Peck observed in 2009, "and yet that time in our history affects our attitudes toward alcohol to this very day" (p. 7).

Prohibition's persistent legacy can be seen in the reaction of a representative of the Drug Policy Alliance to the Oglala Sioux Tribe's policy of prohibiting alcohol at Pine Ridge. This representative wrote on the *Huffington Post*: "As terrible as alcohol and other drugs are for some people, prohibition is not the answer. It didn't work in the United States in the 1920s and it is not working for the Sioux people today" (Newman, 2012). Instead, the representative emphasized the need for greater economic opportunities and more substance abuse prevention programs. The importance of historical experience and pervasive inherited wisdom—correct or not—in shaping contemporary debates about alcohol policy is discussed in depth in Chapter 4.

Regardless of the outcome of the Oglala Sioux's lawsuit, it is clear that these issues will continue to be debated in the coming years. The case also highlights many of the key kinds of issues that are explored in this book, and shows how debates and decisions about alcohol policies are often made in a multilayered context and are affected by historical, cultural, and external forces. These complexities of alcohol policymaking are explored in several other historical and contemporary case studies from around the world that are presented in this book.

A Note on Terminology

The terminology to describe alcohol-related disorders and harms remains the subject of much debate. The fourth edition of the *Diagnostic and Statistical Manual of Mental Disorders* (DSM-IV), produced by the American Psychiatric

Association (1994), identifies two different disorders related to alcohol: "alcohol abuse" and "alcohol dependence." Alcohol abuse is typically defined as "harmful drinking," or alcohol consumption that has serious detrimental effects on an individual's well-being and on the well-being of others (Dinh-Zaar et al., 1999, p. 610). Examples of such detrimental effects include poorer performance or attendance at work or school, or breaking the law. Alcohol dependence, according to the DSM-IV, involves an individual meeting at least three of seven criteria; these criteria include tolerance, withdrawal symptoms when alcohol is not consumed, and continued consumption of alcohol despite knowing that its use has resulted in physical or psychological harm.

The difficulty of defining alcohol-related disorders is shown by the fact that in the new edition of this manual, the DSM-5, these diagnoses will likely be revised. As the DSM-5 was being prepared for a May 2013 publication date, details of planned changes were debated in the media. Media reports suggested that the DSM-IV's distinction between "abuse" and "dependence" would be dropped in the new edition and replaced with a single "addiction" diagnosis that could be graded "mild," "moderate," or "severe" (Szalavitz, 2012b). These proposed changes prompted much debate among experts (Urbina, 2012). The new diagnosis was praised by some observers for eliminating the "stigmatizing" term "abuse" (Szalavitz, 2012a). However, one critic, exploring the possible new "addiction" diagnosis, pointed out that the term "addict" was itself "stigmatizing" (Frances, 2010). The new criteria also faced the additional criticism that they would label some common patterns of excessive drinking as "addictions" (Thompson, 2012a). As one commentator for the US newsmagazine *Time* argued: "From any perspective, it's absurd to potentially label the 40% of college students who get drunk at least once a month as having 'mild' alcoholism" (Szalavitz, 2012b).

The criteria produced by the American Psychiatric Association, however, are not the only criteria used to classify alcohol-related disorders. The WHO (2004b) has also produced a schema, which is described in the *International Statistical Classification of Diseases and Related Health Problems* (ICD-10) and does not include the term "alcohol abuse." Instead, the ICD-10 distinguishes between "harmful use" (defined as recurrent usage with negative psychological or physical effects), and "dependence" (established based upon a range of criteria, including the compulsion to drink and the presence of tolerance and, when alcohol is not consumed, withdrawal symptoms). Other researchers have employed yet further terms to refer to alcohol-related disorders or harms. Rehm and colleagues (2005, p. 377), for example, have used the broader phrase "alcohol use disorders" to refer to both "alcohol dependence and abuse" (DSM-IV) and "harmful use" (ICD-10). Finally, the term "binge drinking" has also been employed by experts to refer to the consumption of a large amount of alcohol within a short time, thus distinguishing this practice from "regular harmful drinking" (Hatton et al., 2009).

The diversity of terms used in the professional literature—and the continuing evolution of these terms—shows just how difficult it can be to define many of the key concepts explored in this book. Yet policymakers are expected to understand these nuances in order to implement effective policies. In this volume, for simplicity, the term "alcohol misuse" is typically employed rather than the more specific terms advanced by the APA or the WHO. Alcohol misuse is a term that is used more frequently in the UK and is defined as "the use of alcohol for a purpose not consistent with legal or medical guidelines" (BMA Board of Science, 2008, p. vi). Although some readers might prefer more specific alternatives, this term was selected because it covers the wider range of issues explored in this book.

Of course, this volume does not focus on alcohol misuse but on policies to reduce or prevent alcohol misuse. Following Edwards and colleagues (1994), the broad term "alcohol policies" is employed here to refer to the wide range of public health measures that societies have implemented to limit the harms of alcohol, ranging from overall taxation to more targeted policies focusing on reducing alcohol-impaired driving (WHO, 2004a, p. 2).

Finally, since this work focuses on policymaking, it is also important to stress that policymaking is defined here as "the procedures involved in getting an issue on the political agenda; formulating, adopting, and implementing a policy with regard to the issue; and then evaluating the results of the policy" (Sidlow and Henschen, 2009, p. 341). Policymaking is thus considered a multistage, complex process, and these stages are fleshed out in Chapter 3. This book primarily discusses policies and programs that are created by actual legislation, rather than bureaucratic administrative orders.

Acknowledging debates about definitions is important; however, it is equally important not to become so mired in these debates that one cannot move on to the actual issues of interest. As Michael Gossop (2007, p. xiii) observed about drug-related terminology in his classic work *Living with Drugs*: "One cannot please all the readers all the time, and I would rather have tried to look at the issues of drugs and drug taking than at the language which we use to talk about them." This statement could equally be applied to the use of alcohol terminology in this book.

An Outline of this Book

Chapter 2 is directed at readers who have little previous knowledge of alcohol's social harms, or of current research about how to best tackle these harms. This chapter offers an overview of the problems associated with alcohol misuse, and outlines global trends in consumption and the types of mitigation strategies currently employed around the world. Such information has also been covered to different extents in other works, but is presented here as it is essential for understanding the analysis and case studies later in this book.

Chapter 3 describes key policymaking theories that political scientists and other policymaking scholars have advanced, exploring whether these theories offer insight into alcohol policymaking. The limited previous literature on alcohol policymaking is also reviewed in depth.

Chapter 4 discusses the historical, social, and cultural factors that can shape drinking patterns and affect the emergence of alcohol's social harms. Such factors are sometimes overlooked in studies of alcohol's social harms, but they are examined closely here since, in addition to impacting consumption and the emergence of social harms, such factors can also influence alcohol policymaking. Anthropological and historical approaches to alcohol's harms are presented here, to complement the public health approach addressed in Chapter 2 and the political science approaches discussed in Chapter 3.

Chapter 5 explores and compares two case studies of efforts to sharply limit the sale and consumption of alcohol. Although the 13-year Prohibition Era in the US in the early twentieth century has been much-studied by scholars, similar efforts in other countries have received relatively less attention. By examining these two additional case studies, this chapter offers a historical and cross-national perspective on prohibition efforts—and the factors that can lead to prohibition policies' failures.

Chapter 6 looks at case studies of policy ideas in two different countries which aimed to reduce harmful drinking *in general* without instituting prohibition. Drawing on a wealth of previous literature across disciplines, the formulation of these policies is probed to assess the explanatory value of the policymaking theories discussed in Chapter 3.

Chapter 7 focuses on policies that target a specific alcohol-related harm: harmful drinking by young people. By investigating case studies in which opposite policy decisions were made in different countries, the chapter further explores the role of research evidence—as well as political, economic, cultural, and other factors—in alcohol policymaking.

Chapter 8 summarizes and integrates the key findings of the case studies, and also adds new analysis. Specific directions for future research on the under-examined but deeply important issue of alcohol policymaking are proposed.

Chapter 2
Research into Alcohol's Social Harms

More than a century ago, the American psychologist William James pointedly wrote: "Sobriety diminishes, discriminates, and says no; drunkenness expands, unites, and says yes" (2008 [originally published 1902], p. 282). Alcohol's "mystical" hold over human beings which James described is illustrated by the central role it has played in religious practices, social interactions, and family celebrations within various societies throughout history. Archaeological evidence recently unearthed in China suggests that alcoholic mead was brewed as early as 9,000 years ago (Thadeusz, 2009), while wine is depicted in Ancient Egyptian pictographs created around 4,000 B.C. ("Alcohol", 2009, p. 34).

Today, alcohol is one of the world's most popular drugs, consumed by around one third of the current global population (WHO, 2004a). Drinking can offer many pleasurable benefits, such as facilitating socialization and relaxation; however, the misuse or excessive consumption of alcohol is associated with a host of personal and societal harms, and sometimes even with fatal results. For example, in Europe more than a tenth of female deaths and about a quarter of male deaths among 15-to-29-year-olds are related to alcohol consumption (*European strategy* ..., 2011). In the UK specifically, in 2010 more than 8,000 deaths were classified as alcohol-related (Dobson and Owen, 2012). Meanwhile, in the US, in 2009 more than 24,500 deaths were due to alcohol-related causes (excluding homicides) (CDC, 2012b, p. 11). These examples merely scratch the surface, for the range of harms associated with alcohol misuse is vast. In addition to long-term health problems, alcohol plays a role in many traffic deaths, while prenatal exposure to alcohol, as mentioned in the previous chapter, is associated with a range of development deficits.

This chapter offers an overview of alcohol consumption patterns around the world, and is provided for readers who have little previous knowledge of the consequences of—and attempts to reduce—alcohol misuse, as well as readers in need of an overview of recent global research in this area. Many of alcohol's most prominent social harms are described, as well as strategies that have been implemented in various countries to reduce them. This background knowledge is essential for examining issues of alcohol policymaking in Chapter 3 and beyond.

What is Alcohol Misuse?

In the previous chapter, alcohol misuse was defined as "the use of alcohol for a purpose not consistent with legal or medical guidelines" (BMA Board of

Science, 2008, p. vi). But what are these "legal or medical guidelines"? In reality, there is no single measure, with governments and other official bodies advancing many varied recommendations.

One commonly-discussed set of guidelines posits that men should not consume more than 40g of alcohol per day and that women should not consume more than 20g of alcohol, defined as 4 and 2 drinks per day respectively (Directorate-General for Health and Consumer Protection, 2006; The Liver Centre, 2003).[1] Not all countries' health bodies have endorsed this set of recommendations, however, and even a relatively quick survey reveals a bewildering range of often conflicting statements. Different countries have advanced different guidelines, with some nations' health departments promoting daily alcohol limits and other nations' health departments emphasizing weekly limits. Some health departments have advised adults to maintain several alcohol-free days each week, and others recommend that pregnant women and young teenagers not drink at all (International Center for Alcohol Policies, 2010b). In addition to health departments, other experts and organizations in various countries have advanced alternate views and recommendations. Adding to the confusion, the systems for measuring alcohol consumption also vary. In the UK, the official measure is based on units, with one unit being equivalent to a 125ml glass of wine that is 8 percent alcohol by volume (ABV); however, this system has not kept pace with developments in the drinks industry, as wine today can often be 13 percent ABV and is commonly served in a 175ml glass, which would equate to 2.3 units ("How many units …", 2003). In contrast to this unit system, US guidelines and data typically focus on standard drinks. A standard US drink is 14 grams (or 0.6 ounces) of pure alcohol, equivalent to 12 ounces of beer or five ounces of wine (CDC, 2012a).

The fact that a US standard drink is 50 percent larger than a UK unit of alcohol is not only confusing to consumers but also frustrates attempts at comparison, and has prompted calls for a universal measurement and guidelines system (Mulley, 2004, p. 6). There have also been calls for guidelines to be stated more simply and communicated to the public more clearly, as past UK surveys have found that—perhaps unsurprisingly—only a tenth of drinkers measure their consumption in units, and just a quarter "understand the practical implications of what a unit is" (Prime Minister's Strategy Unit, 2004, p. 25). Mindful of these differences, the next section reviews key findings about patterns of alcohol consumption—and, more importantly, patterns of alcohol misuse—around the world.

---

1   The guidelines for women are lower, even for a man and a woman of the same body size, because male bodies contain more water which dilutes alcohol more quickly and reduces its exposure to body organs (US Department of Health and Human Services, 2008). Other contributing factors include women's lower average body size and lower levels of an enzyme that metabolizes alcohol (Insel et al., 2013, pp. 318–19).

Patterns of Alcohol Consumption and Misuse

Although a growing body of data now exists on international drinking patterns and rates of alcohol abuse, attempts at cross-national comparisons face numerous challenges. For example, some countries are believed to have higher rates of unrecorded alcohol consumption—or alcohol consumption that does not appear in official statistics—than others (WHO, 2004a, pp. 15–16). Many popular approaches for surveying populations about alcohol use were developed in western industrialized countries, and it is not clear whether such approaches can be easily adapted to other contexts (Dawson, 2003).

Despite these challenges, international data suggest that, while Middle Eastern countries typically report the lowest rates of consumption (normally explained by the fact that consumption of alcoholic beverages is frowned upon or prohibited in Islam), a wide variety of countries—including Uganda, Luxembourg, the Czech Republic, Ireland, the Republic of Moldova, France, Réunion, Bermuda, and Germany—were reported to have the highest rates in a 2004 WHO report (2004a, p. 12). Europe has the highest per capita consumption of any region in the world; some 55 million Europeans are said to consume dangerous levels of alcohol (AMPHORA, 2010). Globally, men are more likely to drink than women, with the gender gap most pronounced in the Islamic areas of the Eastern Mediterranean and in Southeast Asia (Rehm et al., 2003, p. 151). Even in the UK, on average men consume twice as much alcohol per week than women (BMA Board of Science, 2008, p. 1).

How widespread is alcohol misuse? Grant and colleagues (2004) have reported that 4.7 percent of US adults exhibit symptoms of "alcohol abuse"—defined in the previous chapter as alcohol consumption that has serious detrimental effects on an individual's well-being and on the well-being of others (Dinh-Zaar et al., 1999, p. 610). Males and younger people were found to have higher rates of abuse in Grant and colleagues' work.

Of course, in addition to measuring *consumption levels* it is also essential to consider *drinking patterns* (Rehm, Chisholm, et al., 2006). Individuals who have low overall levels of consumption, but who consume alcohol in rare binges, can also experience adverse health consequences. Researchers have long noted vast differences in the "typical" drinking patterns of various societies, or subgroups within societies. The influence of history and culture on the development of these drinking patterns is explored in Chapter 4.

Although the question of what causes alcohol misuse has long occupied researchers, no single, overarching answer has been found. As the Institute of Alcohol Studies (2010, p. 3) has reported: "Research has failed to show that 'problem drinkers' share some common pre-existing psychological or physical abnormality which distinguishes them from the rest of the population." Nevertheless, studies of twins have suggested that around 50 percent of one's risk of developing a *dependence on alcohol* is inherited (Prescott, 2003). Ginter and Simko (2009) have surveyed the wide range of biological mechanisms—such as variations in genes that encode the enzymes used to metabolize alcohol in the human body—that are potentially linked with the development of alcohol abuse.

As Le Strat and colleagues' (2008) review shows, although research has repeatedly found a relationship between alcohol abuse and several variants within GABA receptor genes, the overall relationship between genes and the development of harmful drinking patterns is not straightforward. For example, it has been determined that some people of Asian descent possess a specific genetic polymorphism believed to offer protective effects against the development of alcoholism, and research suggests that members of *some* Native American tribes do not possess this same polymorphism (Elders, 2007). Native Americans have the highest alcohol-related mortality rates of any ethnic group in the US (McFarland et al., 2006; National Institute on Alcohol Abuse and Alcoholism, 2007). However, members of other Native American tribes *have* been found to possess alternative gene polymorphisms believed to offer a protective effect against alcoholism, and these tribes still have high rates of alcohol abuse (Elders, 2007). Indeed, according to the National Institute on Alcohol Abuse and Alcoholism (2007, p. 3), "research shows that there is no difference in the rates of alcohol metabolism and enzyme patterns between Native Americans and Whites"—further highlighting the importance of environmental, sociological, and other non-genetic factors in the development of harmful drinking behaviors.

One final complexity to consider is the finding that genes which seem to offer a protective effect against alcoholism may also, counter-intuitively, increase the chances of developing alcohol-related cancers; since these genes impede the metabolization of alcohol, they leave a drinker exposed to higher levels of acetaldehyde, which may be carcinogenic (National Institute on Alcohol Abuse and Alcoholism, 2007, p. 3; Seitz and Becker, 2007).

This brief overview cannot do justice to the full range of important findings that have emerged about the interplay of genetic and biological factors in the development of harmful drinking practices. However, even this abbreviated summary illustrates the dangers of making generalizations due to the complexity and ever-evolving nature of findings in this area.

Much valuable research has explored the *correlates* and *predictors* of alcohol misuse. In men, predictors of developing problematic patterns of alcohol use include a family history of alcoholism, greater levels of alcohol consumption, and past use of other kinds of drugs (Schuckit, Smith, and Landi, 2000). This third predictor—past use of other kinds of drugs—highlights the importance of also considering other kinds of substance use alongside alcohol misuse. Indeed, according to Staines and colleagues (2001), more than two-thirds of a sample of alcoholics seeking treatment at one New York City hospital said that they had also consumed illicit drugs during the past 90 days, with powder cocaine the most frequently-selected illicit drug. Such behavior is known as polysubstance abuse—in this case, the misuse of both alcohol *and* illicit drugs. Since so many users of illicit drugs also consume excessive amounts of alcohol, alcohol can be a comfounding factor in many studies of the effects of illicit drug use (Fernández-Serrano et al., 2010). Moreover, polysubstance abuse can aggravate the memory deficits and other negative effects associated with alcohol misuse on its own (Bondi, Drake, and Grant, 1998), thus increasing potential social harms. In addition to illicit drugs, research has also highlighted the problem of combining of *prescription drugs* with alcohol use, particularly by older people (Stevenson, 2005).

Drug use is just one potential correlate of alcohol misuse. A second is prenatal exposure to alcohol. Baer and colleagues (2003, pp. 382–3) found that "prenatal alcohol exposure is significantly associated with alcohol-related problems assessed in offspring at 21 years of age," even when accounting for demographics, gender, "family history of alcohol problems," and other potential confounding factors. This finding hints at a potential "vicious cycle" of harmful drinking behaviors, where alcohol misuse by parents can potentially contribute to later alcohol misuse by their grown children.

One final correlate of alcohol misuse to discuss here is mental health issues. Much research has explored alcohol misuse among individuals suffering from post-traumatic stress disorder (Amaro et al., 2007; Kaysen et al., 2006; Kofoed, Friedman, and Peck, 1993)—just one sub-area of research within the much larger literature on the co-occurrence of alcohol use disorders and other mental health issues. However, the relationships between alcohol misuse and mental health issues can be deeply complex. For example, depression can contribute to the development of alcohol abuse, but excessive alcohol consumption can also worsen depression (Pompili et al., 2010). Such complexities highlight the difficulties of identifying causal pathways in this area, and the importance of recognizing the frequent intersection of alcohol and mental health issues when developing treatment and prevention programs.

Trends and Predictions

Total global consumption of alcohol—and the social harms related to consumption—will likely increase in future years, as economic growth in countries like India and China creates more demand (Harrell, 2009; Rehm, Patra, et al., 2006; Rehm et al., 2009). In the US during the 1990s, alcohol abuse and alcohol dependence rates among males both increased (Grant et al., 2004). In recent decades, enthusiasm for free markets and free trade—and the corresponding weakening of many trade barriers and state controlled alcohol retail monopolies—has increased the availability of alcohol in many countries (Jernigan et al., 2000).

Of course, sweeping generalizations about national trends in alcohol consumption do not capture more nuanced changes. During the 2000s, alcohol consumption in the UK actually fell slightly and, despite increased concern about youth drinking in the UK, in 2010 Britain's National Health Service (NHS) reported that more than half of British 11-to-15-year-olds had never consumed alcohol—a higher percentage than in previous years (de Castella, 2012). Yet the mid 2000s also witnessed an increase in the proportion of British young teenagers drinking to get drunk, with more than a third of 11-to-15-year-olds who had drunk alcohol in the previous month before the study was conducted reporting they had done so with the intention of becoming intoxicated (Department for Children, Schools and Families et al., 2008, p. 8). Indeed, cross-national survey data indicate that British teenagers are more likely to report being drunk in the past month than teenagers from almost all other European countries (Smithers, 2009). These findings illustrate the challenges inherent in making general conclusions about trends in drinking. A further complication is the fact that *reactions* to drinking also change over time. As Thom (2007, p. 247) has argued, immediately after World War II, concerns about youth drinking were not very prominent in Britain, yet in the 1980s, such concerns grew alongside the frequency of media reports about youth violence and "lager louts." Today, graphic descriptions of "binge Britain" pervade the media and likely fuel public concern about alcohol (p. 252).

Drinking patterns can change across generations, and such changes can sharply impact trends in overall societal consumption. Härkönen and Mäkelä (2011, p. 349), for example, have detailed how Finnish alcohol consumption levels waxed and waned throughout the past 50 years, with increases sometimes following reductions in alcohol regulations or taxes. Kim and colleagues (2008) also found generational differences in drinking patterns in Hong Kong, which were potentially due to larger demographic and social changes. Documenting longer-term changes in consumption or drinking patterns—i.e., changes that span more than a few decades—presents a greater challenge, due to the paucity of available evidence and data. Interestingly, a large-scale study of young people's drinking patterns was conducted in Austria in the very early twentieth century, which allowed scholars many decades later to compare that data with more recent findings and conclude that alcohol consumption levels among adolescents were very similar in 1900 and 1975 (Lesch et al., 2011, p. 37).

More broadly, Rorabaugh's (2003) synthesis of historical studies of US alcohol consumption reveals that, on average, Americans aged 15 and over consumed 6 gallons of alcohol per person per year during the Colonial Era, although the difficulty of securing reliable data from the period means that this figure is only an estimate. By 1825, average consumption had risen to 7 gallons per person per year, but in the mid-to-late nineteenth century, as the temperance movement gained momentum, consumption fell to about 2 gallons. During the Prohibition Era, according to Rorabaugh, consumption fell to its lowest point of less than 1 gallon, but following the repeal of the Volstead Act it rose again to 2.8 gallons in 1980, settling at 2.2 gallons by 1998. These findings suggest that levels of alcohol consumption are far from constant and can change in response to societal, environmental, and a myriad of other factors.

Alcohol's Long-Term Health Effects

As explained in Chapter 1, this volume employs Room's (2000, p. 94) definition of *social harm* as a "perceived misperformance or failure to perform in major social roles — as a family member, as a worker, as a friend or neighbour, or in terms of public demeanour," which can occur either at a particular moment, or over time. It would be impossible to describe all of alcohol misuse's potential social harms in this chapter. Nevertheless, this section outlines some of the most prominent of these harms, focusing on those that illustrate the range of social problems that alcohol is associated with, as well as those harms that have received the greatest attention from researchers. Readers interested in more comprehensive discussions of alcohol's social harms—and methods to prevent such harms—can refer to Babor and colleagues' (2003) *Alcohol: No Ordinary Commodity* or to the WHO's (2004a) *Global Status Report on Alcohol*. These are just two of the many excellent and more detailed overviews of information in this area.

The first significant social harm to be explored is the set of long-term health risks that alcohol misuse can pose to drinkers. Awareness of such risks dates back centuries, as Benjamin Rush, the American physician discussed in Chapter 1, first linked pneumonia and tuberculosis to alcohol abuse in the 1780s (Ferentzy, 2001); some of these associations that have since been confirmed by contemporary research (Lönnroth et al., 2008; Rehm et al., 2009; Szabo et al., 1997). Today, researchers have found that alcohol plays a causal role in more than 60 kinds of different medical conditions (Room et al., 2005). About 9 percent of Europe's total disease burden is related to alcohol (Rehn, Room, and Edwards, 2001, p. 1), and an estimated 30,000 deaths in the UK each year are alcohol-related (Mulley, 2004, p. 5). Alcohol is the third most significant cause of disease in the developed world—with disease defined as number of years lost due to death or disability—and only tobacco and hypertension are more significant (Babor et al., 2003). Heavy drinking and mortality are significantly related, according to one meta-analysis (Leino et al., 1998, p. 216). A large-scale study of data from 15 European countries from the 1950s to the 1990s found a relationship between higher rates of alcohol consumption in countries and increased alcohol-related mortality (Ramstedt, 2002).

Perhaps the best-known long-term health consequence of excessive alcohol consumption is liver disease, from which over 15,000 Americans die each year (CDC, 2012b, p. 38). Another long-term health consequence is cancer—in particular, cancers of the oral cavity, throat, voice box, and esophagus (Pöschl and Seitz, 2004; Seitz and Becker, 2007). Indeed, more than a fifth of esophageal cancers are due to alcohol consumption (as cited in WHO, 2004, p. 1). In addition, a meta-analysis by Bagnardi and colleagues (2001) found positive, statistically-significant relationships between alcohol consumption and the development of stomach, colon, ovarian, and rectal cancers. Another meta-analysis by Smith-Warner and colleagues (1998) found a positive association between alcohol consumption and breast cancer in women.

Research attention has not only focused on the negative outcomes of alcohol consumption. The question of whether moderate or low alcohol consumption may have some health benefits has also received significant attention in recent years. Low levels of alcohol consumption—even as low as one drink each week—may reduce the chance of stroke (Berger et al., 1999). In a landmark study Thun and colleagues (1997) found that, for adult men and women, rates of cardiovascular diseases were 30–40 percent lower among those who reported consumption of at least one alcoholic drink per week relative to abstainers (heavy drinkers, however, had a higher overall risk of mortality). A systematic review of prospective cohort studies by Ronksley and colleagues (2011) found that light and moderate drinkers had a lower risk of various cardiovascular ailments, as well as a lower risk of overall mortality, than abstainers. However, this review's findings conflicted with the results from earlier research (Leino et al., 1998), and generated significant debate, with some scholars critiquing the limitations of the studies included in the review (Stockwell et al., 2012) and the authors responding (Ronskley et al., 2012).

The British Heart Foundation (2012) responded to findings about moderate consumption's potential benefits by advising that "we would not advise you to start drinking if you don't already" and, within the same document, pointing out that excessive alcohol consumption can contribute to high blood pressure and heart muscle damage. Jernigan and colleagues (2000, p. 492) have also noted that moderate drinking's benefits would likely be small in the developing world, as rates of coronary heart disease are already relatively low in many developing countries.

Costs of Alcohol Consumption

In addition to its terrible human costs, alcohol misuse also poses serious economic costs to developed and developing societies alike. In 1860, a judge in Washington, DC, estimated that alcohol abuse cost the United States "more than *one hundred millions of dollars*" (sic) each year (as reported in Cocker, 1860, p. 9). Some 140 years later, the National Institute on Alcohol Abuse and Alcoholism reported the annual costs were more than $180 billion (Harwood, 2000). The American figures are not unique; Collins and Lapsley (2008) have estimated the annual costs associated with alcohol consumption in Australia to be more than $15.3 billion AUD (equivalent to around $13 billion USD), nearly double that for illicit drugs. Globally, alcohol abuse costs high-income and middle-income countries more than one percent of gross national product (Rehm et al., 2009). One social harm for which the economic costs have been repeatedly estimated is fetal alcohol syndrome (Navarro, Doran, and Shakeshaft, 2011). Stade and colleagues (2009) have estimated that, in Canada, the annual per-individual cost of treating this single harm alone is more than $21,000 CAD (equivalent to more than $18,400 billion USD).

The question of how to best estimate the society-wide costs of alcohol consumption has prompted much debate. Many estimates of alcohol's costs have focused solely on harms to the individual drinkers themselves, but not on alcohol's harms to others, thus potentially underestimating the true cost burden of alcohol (Navarro et al., 2011). On the other hand, in a provocative working paper Crampton and Burgess (2009) criticized examples of cost estimates that did not take into account the health benefits of moderate drinking and that assumed that, if not for alcohol, chronic excessive drinkers would otherwise participate in the labor force in similar ways to non-excessive drinkers. According to the authors, these and other oversights could lead to *overestimations* of alcohol's social costs.

Another factor that can further complicate efforts to estimate alcohol's impact is the fact that, through taxes, alcohol can generate significant *revenue* for governments. The Thai government, for example, gains almost 6 percent of its net income from alcohol excise taxes, according to 2005 data (Thamarangsi, 2008, p. 5). (On the other hand, the health, criminal justice, and other costs of alcohol consumption are equivalent to nearly 2 percent of that country's annual GDP [Thavorncharoensap et al., 2010]). To generate revenue during the economic recession that began in 2008, a number of US states and cities loosened alcohol retail restrictions but raised alcohol taxes—however some critics worried this strategy could be counterproductive in the long run if alcohol's social harms increased (Severson, 2011). Although, in many societies, alcohol's costs outweigh these revenues, income as well as expenditure must be taken into account for a complete understanding of alcohol's economic impact.

The Public Health Approach

Physicians and other medical experts have long studied the effects of excessive alcohol consumption. Indeed, as described in Chapter 1, Benjamin Rush pioneered the idea of "addiction" to alcohol in the 1780s and 1790s (Butterfield, 1950; Ferentzy, 2001), while the American Medical Association first classified alcoholism as a disease in the 1950s (Mersy, 2003). In contemporary times, the public health approach to alcohol issues—which focuses on trying to prevent or mitigate health issues that arise from alcohol consumption in the overall population—has gained increasing prominence. In 1975, the landmark volume *Alcohol Control Policies in Public Health Perspective* was published under the auspices of the World Health Organization (WHO). This volume—lead-authored by the Finnish public health pioneer Kettil Bruun—marked the ascendancy of the public health perspective (see Room, 1984, for a discussion of this time period). Bruun and his co-authors argued that, given the relationship between alcohol consumption and health issues in society, controlling the availability of alcohol could be considered a *public health* priority (p. 13). The volume signaled the ascendancy of an increasingly internationalized approach to researching and mitigating alcohol's social harms. Interestingly, as Tigerstedt (1999; citing Bruun, 1971) has detailed, on a personal level Bruun was concerned that policies which singled out and aimed to control "problematic" drinkers could be deeply discriminatory; instead, Bruun believed that population-level policies—such as raising the price of alcohol or limiting alcohol advertising—would be less stigmatizing and more effective.

Today the WHO—through its Global Strategy discussed in Chapter 1 and other influential works—and many public health experts tirelessly highlight the health impacts of excessive drinking and promote the idea that the public should be informed about alcohol's risks. In doing so, they continue to work in the vein of the American Revolutionary-era physician Benjamin Rush who, as described in Chapter 1, shared these two goals (Katcher, 1993). Health organizations *within* many countries also conduct important contemporary research in this area. In the US, for example, the National Institute on Alcohol Abuse and Alcoholism (NIAAA)—a research institute within the National Institutes of Health (NIH)— was founded in 1970, and by 2008 operated with a budget of $439 million, much of which was devoted to research (Kastor, 2010, p. 90). In Europe, the Alcohol Measures for Public Health Research Alliance (AMPHORA), a major public health research initiative, was set into motion in 2009; it will cost an estimated €4 million and its studies will span at least a dozen different countries (Gual and Anderson, 2012; König and Segura, 2011).

Within the public health approach, a number of important sub-perspectives have emerged which attempt to conceptualize alcohol's social harms. The first of these, the social determinants of health perspective, emphasizes the environmental, physical, and other social conditions that can affect individuals' health outcomes and life trajectories (WHO, 2012c). Advocates of this perspective stress that public health problems are often a partial result of—or are exacerbated by—political, economic, social, and other larger factors. International power dynamics can also play a role. Of particular concern are the impacts of poverty and economic inequality on health and wellness disparities in populations (British Medical Association, 2011). The WHO (2011a) has emphasized the importance of considering these determinants when targeting alcohol's social harms, writing in its alcohol factsheet: "The health, safety and socioeconomic problems attributable to alcohol can be effectively reduced and requires actions on the levels, patterns and contexts of alcohol consumption and the wider *social determinants of health*" (emphasis added).

A second sub-perspective that needs to be examined here is the harm reduction approach. Originally developed in response to illicit drugs' social harms—and, in particular, the spread of HIV through drug injection needles (Carter, Miller, and Hall, 2012, p. 111)—the harm reduction approach has been increasingly applied to alcohol (Müller, 2004, p. 2). This approach focuses on reducing the social harms that can result from the use of a drug (in this case, alcohol) without necessarily endeavoring to also reduce overall consumption or to reduce consumption that does not result in harms (Marlatt and Witkiewitz, 2002). The harm reduction approach to alcohol can be seen in the European Commission's 2006 alcohol strategy, which "specifically targets the harmful and hazardous effects of alcohol consumption rather than the product itself. The objective is to reduce the damage caused by this *kind* of alcohol consumption" (*European strategy …*, 2011) (emphasis added).

The logic behind the harm-reduction approach can be seen in the arguments of a Malaysian commentator, quoted at the beginning of Chapter 1: "Alcohol consumption will not stop, and what policymakers must concentrate on is changing the environment so persons who consume alcohol do not drink excessively, and that they are protected from alcohol-related harm" (Rahman, 2012). Advocates of the harm reduction approach argue that since significantly reducing alcohol consumption itself is not feasible, governments' limited resources should instead target alcohol-impaired driving, long-term excessive consumption, and other potentially harmful types of alcohol use.

Initiatives to Reduce Alcohol's Harms

How can societies best reduce the harms associated with alcohol? Should governments adopt the perspective of Kettil Bruun (1971)—the public health expert described in the previous section—and adopt population-level policies, such as price increases or restrictions on advertising, so as not to discriminate against individual subsets of drinkers? Or should governments instead adopt a harm reduction approach and target specific problems rather than overall consumption? Is it desirable—or even possible—for governments to take into account the social determinants of health when formulating alcohol policies? Regardless of how one answers these questions, it is clear that devising policies to most effectively reduce alcohol's social harms is a mammoth task. This section offers a short overview of the different kinds of policies that societies have adopted, or could adopt. Key research evidence about the effectiveness of these policies is also presented. Many different kinds of policies have been trialed to combat alcohol's harms and not all such policies could be discussed here. Instead, this section's overview offers the essential background information required for the examination of the case studies in future chapters.

Policies for controlling alcohol use and reducing alcohol's social harms are about as old as alcohol abuse itself. More than 3,700 years ago the Ancient Babylonian Code of Hammurabi established regulations governing the sale of alcohol, whilst, at various points in the histories of Ancient Greece, Rome, and Persia, efforts were made to decrease excessive drinking (Youngerman, 2005, p. 23). Debates about whether wine promoted or harmed health were rife in Renaissance Europe (Albala, 2006), and both Protestant and Catholic reformers railed against drunkenness in the post-Reformation period (Holt, 2006). In England in 1552, a formal licensing system for alehouses—overseen by Justices of the Peace—was enacted to combat drunkenness and related harms, as well as to target a key breeding ground for social unrest (London Metropolitan Archives, 1998). In the US, taxes on various alcoholic beverages have been imposed since the country's earliest days (Cook, 2007). The growth of temperance movements in many countries in the nineteenth and early twentieth centuries led to increasing restrictions on alcohol. Most famously, the American temperance movement encouraged the passage of the Eighteenth Amendment (via the Volstead Act), which outlawed the manufacture and sale of alcohol; the Eighteenth Amendment was ratified in 1919 but its prohibition of alcohol was repealed in 1933 (Hamm, 1995). The consequences of instituting prohibition policies are described in more detail in Chapter 5.

Today the simplest and most common policy that governments employ to reduce alcohol's social harms is taxation. By increasing the price for alcohol, policymakers typically aim to decrease overall alcohol consumption and therefore reduce alcohol's social harms. A meta-analysis by Wagenaar, Salois, and Komro (2009) examined the relationship between alcohol taxes and prices and consumption, drawing on 112 studies. The meta-analysis found that higher prices were associated with lower alcohol consumption, and this relationship held true for beer, wine, and spirits. Higher prices were associated with lower consumption by both low-level and high-level drinkers. Other research promisingly indicates that adolescent drinking habits might be more responsive to increases in the price of alcohol (Xu and Chaloupka, 2011). Additionally, there is evidence that in Finland in 2004, introducing the opposite policy—a reduction in alcohol excise taxes—was followed by an increase in alcohol-related deaths (Mäkelä and Osterberg, 2009).

More generally, some public health experts have expressed concern at the relatively low prices of alcohol beverages in some countries. For example, Gunasekara and Wilson (2010) reported that, in New Zealand, a bottle of beer or a glass of wine sometimes cost less than a glass of bottled water and only a little bit more than a glass of milk. Xu and Chaloupka (2011) observed that US federal and state excise taxes on alcohol have only been subject to rare increases and consequently have fallen substantially in real monetary terms. Concerns about low prices for alcohol leading to greater social harms prompted the Scottish Parliament to adopt a minimum price of 50 pence per unit of alcohol in 2012 (Carrell, 2012). When policymakers debate increasing alcohol taxes, it is important for them to also consider what the revenue generated by those taxes will be used for. Müller (2004, p. 2) has pointed out that countries often place the revenue generated from alcohol taxes into a general fund, rather than specifically using it to fight alcohol's social harms. According to Müller, this practice can cause the public to view such taxes as simply additional revenue-generating measures for governments, rather than as harm mitigation strategies—further eroding public support for these policies.

In some countries and regions, governments do not merely tax alcohol—they maintain a monopoly on its manufacture and sale. For example, after Prohibition was repealed in the US in 1933, several US states instituted government monopolies and, to this day, seven states retain such systems, while an eighth state, Washington, transitioned from a monopoly to a private system in 2012 (Johnson, 2012). Parts of Canada and the entire country of Sweden also maintain government alcohol monopolies (de Castella, 2012). Monopoly systems allow governments to collect more revenue and, with their typically understated displays, monopoly-owned stores do not encourage consumption in the way that many private stores do (de Castella, 2012; Johnson, 2012). A 2010 study by Norström and colleagues projected that, in Sweden, replacing the alcohol monopoly with private stores would lead to a 17 percent increase in alcohol consumption, as well as over 8,000 more assaults each year. Other policies societies have instituted to restrict the sale of alcohol include instituting a minimum age for purchases, limiting the trading hours of alcohol retail outlets, and maintaining a rigorously-enforced licensing system to sell alcohol; all three of these strategies are supported by a strong or moderate evidence base (Babor et al., 2003). On the other hand, not all policies to reduce alcohol misuse are supported by research evidence. For example, although educational campaigns about alcohol's harms often enjoy public support and seem to increase public knowledge about these harms, they do not always affect public drinking habits (Parry, 2005).

In addition to the measures described above, other policies and programs focus more specifically on those drinkers with high levels of consumption. Reaching heavy, persistent, and problematic drinkers—whether young or old—poses numerous challenges. One approach that can be beneficial is to encourage physicians to offer brief advice to their patients who misuse alcohol (Mersy, 2003). Indeed, a WHO-sponsored project that featured counseling sessions with health professionals and which was trialed in Australia, Kenya, Mexico, Norway, Russia, the UK, the US, and Zimbabwe obtained promising results (WHO Brief Intervention Study Group, 1996). As Dongier (2003) has noted, alcohol abuse is one of the most common disorders physicians must deal with, so the importance of encouraging physicians to offer advice to alcohol-misusing patients should not be underestimated.

Perhaps the best-known method for helping individuals cease problematic drinking behaviors is the 12-step program of Alcoholics Anonymous (AA), which began in the US in the 1930s and has now spread around the world (Martin, 2008). In AA, alcoholics come together to share their stories and help each other, with the goal of achieving sobriety (Walker, 1989). The issue of how to best evaluate the effectiveness of AA and other 12-step programs has generated much controversy (e.g., Kaskutas, 2008). A Cochrane Collaboration systematic review of studies of AA and other twelve-step programs identified a need for more rigorous, experimental evaluations (Ferri et al., 2006). In another review, Kaskutas (2009, p. 155) concluded that: "Among the rigorous experimental studies, there were two positive findings for AA effectiveness, one null finding and one negative finding." The dearth of evidence could be in part due to the particular difficulties of overcoming selection bias in evaluating a voluntary program—difficulties that some researchers have attempted to overcome through statistical methods (Kaskutas, 2009). Additionally, establishing the reasons why individuals drop out of AA in studies of the program's effectiveness can be challenging (Sharma and Branscum, 2010, p. 5), perhaps due to the importance of anonymity in the program. Nevertheless, despite these mixed findings and methodological challenges, many public health experts agree that alcoholics who seek help from AA have more positive outcomes than those who do not seek help at all (see Babor et al., 2003, pp. 215–16, for a discussion of the relevant literature).

Targeted strategies have also been developed to reduce specific harms associated with alcohol misuse. For example, minimum drinking age policies have been developed to reduce the specific problem of underage drinking. Such policies are discussed in depth in Chapter 7.

Conclusion

No single chapter—indeed, no single book—can offer a comprehensive international overview of alcohol consumption and policies to reduce alcohol's harms. The aim of this chapter has been to present information essential for analyzing the policies and case studies described later in this volume. The harms discussed in this chapter were selected because of their societal importance, their prominence in the literature, and the availability of informative related case studies.

The examination of alcohol's social harms presented in this chapter was, of course, very *general*. Yet even this very general discussion revealed that very specific factors—such as historical, cultural, and other characteristics—can affect societies' drinking practices and determine which alcohol-related policies are adopted. These differences mean that not all policies to reduce alcohol's social harms will be effective everywhere. Some policies and programs discussed in this chapter—such as higher taxes on alcohol—are not culturally-specific and have a diverse evidence base that suggests they could work in many contexts (Babor et al., 2010). For other policies, however, more consideration is needed before transferring them to different countries and new cultural contexts. Indeed, researchers have found cross-national differences in the most effective strategies to combat alcohol misuse. For example, according to Chisholm and colleagues (2004), more targeted approaches such as encouraging family doctors to educate at-risk patients about the hazards of alcohol abuse seem to be more cost-effective in low-consumption countries, while higher taxation is highly cost-effective in countries with high levels of alcohol consumption. The importance of such cross-national nuances is a theme that is revisited throughout this book and is discussed in detail in Chapter 4.

This chapter focused on what is perhaps the most prevalent contemporary framework for theorizing about alcohol's social harms: the public health perspective. However, insights from other disciplines are also essential for understanding the alcohol policymaking process, and crafting effective alcohol policies. In the next chapter, relevant findings from political science are reviewed in detail, while Chapter 4 explores anthropological and historical ideas that can aid policy development and implementation. Although the harms discussed in this chapter have been discussed in many past reviews, this book builds on these past discussions and brings together the insights of other disciplines and historical case studies to effectively combat these harms.

Chapter 3
Alcohol and Policymaking

What factors influence the alcohol policymaking process? This chapter draws upon key theories from the general policymaking and political science literatures to answer this question and to develop a theoretical base from which to explore real-world case studies of alcohol policymaking. These case studies, discussed in Chapter 4 and beyond, illuminate the explanatory value and the limitations of these theories, and thereby identify important directions for future research in this area.

In Chapter 1, policymaking was defined as a multistage process comprising "the procedures involved in getting an issue on the political agenda; formulating, adopting, and implementing a policy with regard to the issue; and then evaluating the results of the policy" (Sidlow and Henschen, 2009, p. 341). Policymaking is thus a complex undertaking with constituent parts that must be examined; indeed, sub-processes such as agenda-setting—or how policies come to the attention of policymakers in the first place (Kingdon, 2003)—are explored in depth in this chapter. Additionally, as the international transfer of alcohol policies is becoming increasingly prevalent in the globalized world, the question of why some policies spread across countries and regions is also examined. Although surprisingly few previous studies have explored alcohol policymaking *specifically*, the findings of this important body of research are outlined at the end of this chapter.

Inevitably, only a selection of the many theories of policymaking that scholars have advanced can be examined here. The theories from the general policymaking literature that are discussed in this chapter were selected because they are among the most prominent frameworks in the general literature. They also have the greatest potential for explaining alcohol-related policy decisions as evidenced by their application in previous alcohol-related studies; such applications are discussed in detail below.

The Role of Evidence

General knowledge about evidence's role in policymaking has increased markedly in recent years, as public rhetoric about "evidence-based policies" has ballooned. However, theories about the role of evidence in policymaking are by no means new. Indeed, the most influential optimistic vision of how evidence could impact policy was advanced more than 60 years ago by the American political scientist Harold D. Lasswell (1951).

Policy Orientation

Lasswell argued that a "policy orientation" in the social sciences—or an increased interest among social scientists in the nuances of policymaking and the development of better evidence to aid policy decisions—would improve policies. Lasswell's belief that the systematic application of knowledge and evidence could help ameliorate social problems has been revived in more recent times among advocates of the evidence-based policymaking movement. Such advocates, to quote Parsons (2002, p. 45), believe they can "move policy-making ... to a new firm ground" where it will be "driven by evidence, rather than political ideology or prejudice." To cite one famous example, some vanguards of New Labour's 1997 electoral victory in the UK expressed great enthusiasm for evidence-based policymaking and greater cooperation between researchers and policymakers— yet at least one scholar has since expressed disappointment at the actual amount of evidence-based policymaking that took place during New Labour's years in power (Stevens, 2007).

Two Communities

A second major framework for understanding the role of evidence in policymaking stands in sharp contrast to Lasswell's optimistic vision. This framework, known as the "two communities" thesis, posits that researchers and policymakers come from fundamentally different worlds and hence have difficulty communicating and working together to achieve policy goals (Rich, 1991, p. 324; Dunn, 1980). According to this thesis, social scientists and other researchers are thought to be "concerned with 'pure' science and esoteric issues," whilst policymakers "are action-oriented, practical persons concerned with obvious and immediate issues" (Caplan, 1979, p. 459). These differences in motivations, values, and languages make it difficult for researchers to understand policymakers' perspectives, and vice versa—thus impeding collaboration and meaningful debate (Innvaer et al., 2002). Policymakers often seek evidence that is presented concisely and clearly addresses a pressing and relevant problem (Brownson, Chriqui, and Stamatakis, 2009); the nuanced and limited findings from many research studies, however, do not offer straightforward answers. Frustratingly, the difficulties of facilitating communication between the two communities of policymakers and researchers are compounded by the complexity of the policymaking process and the fact that no central coordinator oversees the interactions between different groups of stakeholders (Lindblom, 1979). Ultimately, although Dunn (1980, p. 515) has asserted that the "two communities" framework should perhaps be considered a "metaphor" rather than a "theory," since it is not easily testable and does not aim to explain all aspects of policymaking, this "metaphor" still offers a salient—if pessimistic—perspective.

Specific Circumstances

A third set of ideas, found in the work of Carol H. Weiss (1982), constitute a vision of policymaking that occupies the middle-ground between Lasswell's optimism and "two communities" pessimism. Weiss' work posits that evidence *can* impact policy, but only in certain ways and under specific circumstances. For example, the level of democracy in a country, the amount of centralization in policymaking, and the professional backgrounds of policymakers themselves could all affect the role that evidence and evaluation play in policy decisions (Weiss, 1999, pp. 480–82). Additionally, although the findings of one particular study are unlikely to significantly affect policy, the *general ideas* that emerge from a field can influence discourse. As Weiss (1982, pp. 620–21) explained: "Rarely does research supply an 'answer' that policy actors employ to solve a policy problem. Rather, research provides a background of data, empirical generalizations, and ideas that affect the way that policy makers think about problems." These overarching background ideas might be more influential than an individual study's detailed findings.

Support for the idea that research *can* influence policy under specific circumstances, and at particular moments in time, can be found in Kingdon's (2003) theory of agenda-setting. A landmark theory in political science (Krehbiel, 1998), it aims to explain how and why particular policies rise onto policymakers' agendas. According to Kingdon, in order for policies to receive attention from policymakers, such policymakers must first identify that a "problem" exists. Additionally, relevant stakeholders, such as government officials, scholars, members of pressure groups or other interested parties must put forward a policy "solution" that might ameliorate this problem (p. 87). Finally, a political climate that is supportive of the conservative or liberal nature of the policy also needs to exist for that policy solution to receive serious consideration.

The first of these three steps—when policymakers recognize that a problem exists—offers an opportunity for evidence to influence policy. According to Kingdon, policymakers often recognize the existence of a problem through "indicators," such as statistics and studies that "assess the magnitude of a problem" and help those in power recognize that a problem has worsened (p. 91).[1] Therefore, according to Kingdon's framework, presenting statistical research evidence about the magnitude of alcohol's social harms could help alcohol policies rise onto the political agenda.

Additionally, the second of Kingdon's three steps—the need for bureaucrats, researchers, or others to advance a policy "solution" to the problem—also offers a potential role for research evidence. Policymakers want to attach feasible solutions to problems before they bring those problems onto the legislative agenda (p. 115). Research evidence could thus be used at this point to demonstrate the effectiveness

---

1   In addition to indicators, the second primary way policymakers recognize problems is through "feedback" from the public, such as direct complaints from citizens about a problem (Kingdon, 2003, p. 101).

of a particular policy solution. In particular, Kingdon's framework posits that "policy entrepreneurs" play a key role in advancing policy solutions; these are typically well-connected and committed individuals who can persuasively link policy solutions to pressing problems (pp. 180–82). Policy entrepreneurs can thus be especially important for ensuring that *evidence-based* policy solutions rise onto the legislative agenda.

Although the third step in Kingdon's theory—a sympathetic political climate—does not explicitly include a role for research evidence, this step should not be overlooked by researchers. Since, in Kingdon's framework, a sympathetic political climate is just as important as problem recognition and the advancement of a policy solution, it is essential to pay attention to political factors such as changes in public opinion, influential drives by interest groups, and alterations in legislative partisan balances to seek opportunities to influence evidence-based policymaking.

Competing Interests

In addition to arguing that evidence can influence policy under specific circumstances, Weiss (1983) has also advanced a more general understanding of how competing interests can shape the policymaking process. Unlike Kingdon, who focused on how issues arise onto the legislative agenda, Weiss has examined the policymaking process in general. Specifically, her work has posited that policymaking is shaped by different and competing interests and that power imbalances are fundamental in determining which interests dominate.[2] As power balances shift, the influence of research can also wax and wane. Importantly, Weiss' (1983) insights reveal that research evidence must compete against *other* kinds of "evidence" for policymakers' attention. Such other kinds of "evidence" include the anecdotes, rival claims, and pieces of (sometimes inaccurate) information that other stakeholders advance during the policy process.

Ritter and Bammer (2010, p. 354) have posited that Weiss' ideas can be applied to alcohol-related policymaking by illuminating both the role of interest groups representing the alcohol industry, and the competition between research evidence and other kinds of information in the alcohol policy process. More specifically, Weiss' ideas offer insight into Miller and colleagues' (2011) findings about alcohol policymaking in Australia. Miller and colleagues' studies show that the alcohol industry was influential in promoting strategies that would not significantly harm the industry's profits but would give the appearance that action was being taken against alcohol's social harms. According to their research, such strategies were often promoted at the expense of alternatives, such as higher alcohol taxes, which have a stronger evidence base but *would* harm the industry's profits. Bakke and Endal (2010) have similarly traced the influence of the alcohol industry

---

2   The importance of understanding the distribution of power and the ways in which different stakeholder groups interact has also been emphasized by Brugha and Varvasovszky (2000).

in promoting industry-friendly alcohol policies in four sub-Saharan African countries. Both Miller and colleagues' and Bakke and Endal's findings highlight the validity of Weiss' idea that research evidence must compete with rival claims, and powerful interests.

The influence of Weiss' work—and that of other scholars who wrote on similar themes—can be seen in the shift that took place in the late twentieth century, whereby rational frameworks for understanding policymaking were de-emphasized in favor of theories focusing on the relative power of various actors in the political process. This shift in theoretical perspectives can be seen even in some studies of health-related policymaking (Brugha and Varvasovszky, 2000, p. 240), and likely was in part prompted by the WHO's realization in the late 1970s "that health policymaking did not follow this rational model" and therefore political factors also needed to be studied (Bärnighausen and Bloom, 2011, p. 488).

Incremental Changes

One final idea to consider when exploring the potential influence of evidence on policymaking was advanced by the political scientist Charles E. Lindblom in a now legendary 1959 article. The article's title—"The Science of 'Muddling Through'"—is how Lindblom defined policymaking itself. The framework he advanced in this article, and expanded upon in a 1979 work, is known as "incrementalism" since it posits that policymaking typically consists of small, incremental changes rather than dramatic changes. According to Lindblom, policymakers "muddle through" the intricate process of policymaking, selecting new policies that are similar in many ways to the policies already in place. Policy change therefore typically occurs in small steps rather than revolutionary leaps. Lindblom's conception of policymaking contrasts sharply with the view put forward by advocates of evidence-based policymaking. As Parsons (2002, p. 45) has written, evidence-based policymaking advocates typically believe one can "move policy-making out of the realm of *muddling through* to a new firm ground where policy could be driven by evidence, rather than political ideology or prejudice" (emphasis added). Nevertheless, Lindblom's view of policymaking remains one of the most influential perspectives in political science and is important to consider here. It also provides a useful lens through which to analyze the case studies examined in future chapters.

What Kind of Evidence?

In any examination of evidence-based policymaking, the question of *what constitutes evidence* is fundamental. Although rigorous empirical research is the type of evidence that researchers typically emphasize, it is by no means the only form of evidence presented. Policymakers often also must navigate through a maze of alternative evidentiary sources (Weiss, 1983), including anecdotes and misleading or poorly-conducted studies. Even when rigorous empirical research is offered, policymakers sometimes only "look for evidence to support their claims, and thus systematic bias occurs in the way that policy makers look for and use data" (Choi et al., 2005, p. 633). In policy debates, evidence can sometimes be deployed in a "tactical" manner to serve established interests (Stevens, 2007, p. 31).

Concern about policymakers' tendencies to only select evidence that matches predetermined policy views is at the heart of "Evidence based policy or policy based evidence?", an editorial published in the *BMJ* by a leading epidemiologist (Marmot, 2004). As the editorial points out: "Scientific findings do not fall on blank minds that get made up as a result. Science engages with busy minds that have strong views about how things are and ought to be" (Marmot, 2004, p. 906). Additionally, it must be recognized that all empirical studies have limitations, but policymakers can be concerned that "highlighting knowledge gaps will reduce support for their programmes" (Choi et al., 2005, p. 633), and so might not fully engage with these limitations.

Ultimately, deciding what constitutes evidence in a public health or social scientific context can be a mammoth task. As Manzi (2012, p. xiv) has recently observed, the sheer complexity of human activities makes it "far harder to generalize the results of experiments" in the social sciences than in the natural or physical sciences. This inability to generalize is a significant drawback, since the policies that experiments and evidence seek to inform must be applied in differing areas with different populations. One critic has asserted that "the limited predictive success and the lack of consensus in social sciences" mean that the findings of research "can seldom be primary guides to setting policy" (Gutting, 2012). Other critics have not ventured this far, but have argued that more rigorous research studies—in particular, more randomized trials—are needed to ensure that only high-quality evidence affects policy or practice (Manzi, 2012, p. xvi).

Enthusiasm for randomized controlled trials in the social sciences to determine "what works" can be seen in the well-known work of the development economists Esther Duflo and Abhijit Banerjee (2011), and when researchers talk or write about research influencing policy they often mean this kind of scientific knowledge or evidence. However, as Head (2008) has observed, in addition to "scientific (research-based) knowledge," two other types of knowledge are also relevant for policymaking: "political knowledge" and "practical implementation knowledge" (pp. 5–6). Political knowledge involves insight into how the political system itself operates; in particular, it includes knowledge of how to build coalitions, marshal support, identify a government's goals, and ensure that key messages about a policy are articulated to the public. Practical implementation knowledge includes the know-how of implementing policies and making them "work"; practitioners, bureaucrats, and others with long experience in the field are the principal purveyors of this type of knowledge. Head's emphasis on these two additional kinds of knowledge reminds us of the importance of non-scientific and non-research-determined knowledge in the policymaking process.

So far this section has described various *theoretical* perspectives about the relationship between evidence and policymaking. However, in addition to these outlooks, some *empirical* research has also explored the relationship between evidence and policy. Innvaer and colleagues (2002), for example, systematically reviewed studies that explored policymakers' views on the role of evidence in health-related policymaking. In the 24 studies that met the review's inclusion criteria, the most commonly-cited factor that policymakers identified as facilitating the use of research evidence in policymaking was "personal contact between researchers and policy-makers," whilst "absence of personal contact between researchers and policy-makers" was the most-frequently-cited *impediment* to the use of research evidence (p. 241). Interestingly, this finding corresponds with an idea advanced several decades ago about how to overcome the divide between the "two communities" of researchers and policymakers. Specifically, Caplan (1979, p. 459) wrote that: "Some argue that the gap between the knowledge producer and the policy maker needs to be bridged through personal relationships involving trust, confidence, and empathy." Innvaer and colleagues' findings lend this idea substantial empirical support.

In addition to personal contact, other commonly-cited *facilitating* factors in Innvaer and colleagues' review included "research that included a summary with clear recommendations" and "research that confirmed current policy or endorsed self-interest" (p. 241). The first factor shows the importance of presenting research so it can be easily understood and utilized by policymakers, while the latter factor seems to offer yet more support for Weiss' (1983) idea that competing interests drive policymaking. Indeed, it seems that research evidence's level of influence can depend upon its fit with dominant interests.

On the other hand, Innvaer and colleagues' finding that "mutual mistrust" between research-producers and policymakers was a frequently-cited impediment to using research evidence in policymaking underscores the importance of positive personal relationships between researchers and policy stakeholders. Other commonly-cited impediments included "power and budget struggles" and "political instability or high turnover of policy-making staff" (p. 241), results that support Kingdon's emphasis on political factors in policymaking. One final often-cited impediment in Innaver and colleagues' review was the "poor quality of research." This final finding is also important to consider as it shows that policymakers at least *claim* to be discerning about the quality of evidence that is presented to them.

Policy Diffusion

The theories and frameworks discussed in the previous section all focused on policymaking itself. Yet a second, related process—policy diffusion—is also central to many governments' decisions about alcohol. Policy diffusion is the process by which policies spread from one region or country to another region or country (Karch, 2007; Walker, 1969). Sometimes referred to as policy transfer, this process—and the factors that facilitate the cross-national or cross-regional migration of policies—has been studied by scholars from a range of different disciplines (Allen et al., 2004; Berry, 1994; Jones and Newburn, 2007). As discussed earlier in this chapter, alcohol policy has become increasingly internationalized in recent times, with supranational organizations such as the WHO encouraging the adoption of evidence-based policies. Given this internationalization, understanding how and why certain policies spread internationally is more important than ever.

Dobbin, Simmons, and Garrett's (2007) influential research on policy diffusion offers insight into these issues, as it identifies several key explanations about why policies, practices, and programs diffuse across countries and regions. One such explanation advanced by Dobbin and colleagues is that diffusion is driven by international networks of experts and large global organizations that promote a given set of practices. In the realm of alcohol policymaking, advocates of this explanation would likely seize upon the WHO's (2010) influence in shaping countries' policies through its Global Strategy, as well as the growing impact of collaborative alcohol research by global public health experts.

According to Dobbin and colleagues, a second explanation for why some policies diffuse is the coercive influence of dominant countries and global economic institutions such as the International Monetary Fund (IMF) or World Trade Organization (WTO) on the international stage. Such entities can threaten sanctions against countries that fail to adopt particular policies. For alcohol policies, free trade policies advocated by some supranational organizations can complicate countries' efforts to reduce alcohol's harms by enforcing alcohol import quotas and other trade barriers—an issue explored in detail in a case study in Chapter 6.

One other potentially relevant explanation that Dobbin and colleagues have outlined is that of policy learning. This explanation stresses that countries learn from other's experiences; if one country adopts a policy that seems to be successful, other countries will want to bring that policy to their own territory. Conversely, if one country adopts a policy that seems to be a failure, other countries will be more likely to avoid that approach. The question of whether countries *actually* learn from the policies employed elsewhere is revisited later in this book.

In addition to Dobbin and colleagues' work, one finding from Jack Walker's (1969) seminal early research on policy diffusion is also essential to mention here. Walker found that some US states shared certain characteristics—such as wealth and a large population—which meant that they were consistently more likely to adopt or import new policies than other states (Walker, 1969). The question of whether certain countries or societies are consistent pioneers in regards to alcohol policies, and whether Walker's ideas explain these states' actions, is also important to consider.

In their study of the cross-national diffusion of criminal justice policies from the US to the UK in recent decades, Jones and Newburn (2007) found that particular policymakers and bureaucrats played essential roles in the diffusion process, thus echoing Kingdon's (2003, pp. 180–82) idea that certain individuals—termed "policy entrepreneurs"—can dramatically affect policy choices. Jones and Newburn also found that *rhetoric* about a policy and the problem it targets sometimes diffused more widely than the policy itself. The related idea that rhetoric and language about alcohol and alcohol's social harms can diffuse across countries has been studied by Berridge, Herring, and Thom (2009). Their work has revealed how the term "binge drinking" began to be used in the US to describe excessive drinking among university students—i.e., five drinks in a row for males and four drinks in a row for females. The term subsequently migrated to the UK and is now widely used among British commentators to describe the excessive consumption of alcohol within a very short timeframe.

Returning to the issue of policy diffusion, it is important to recognize that what "works" in one society does not always work when migrated elsewhere, even with local modifications; indeed, policymakers' attempts to adapt policies to meet local conditions are not always successful. Dolowitz and Marsh (2000, p. 17) have identified several key problems that can interfere with policy diffusion and cause imported policies to fail. The first such problem is "uniformed transfer," which involves policymakers and other stakeholders failing to investigate all aspects of the policy under consideration, and not thoroughly examining the setbacks other countries have encountered when implementing that policy. The second problem, according to Dolowitz and Marsh, is "incomplete transfer," or the failure to import *all* aspects of a policy—some of which are essential for the policy to succeed. The third and final problem, "inappropriate transfer," involves policymakers and stakeholders overlooking the fact that a policy was designed to fit a different political or economic system, or was designed to achieve specific goals, which do not apply in the new country. Dolowitz and Marsh's ideas are returned to later in this book, as they offer insight into several of the policymaking case studies.

Research on Alcohol Policymaking

Up until this point, this chapter has focused on the general literature about policymaking, the use of evidence, and the diffusion of policies across borders. The next section, however, looks more specifically at the *alcohol* policymaking literature. Alcohol policymaking has received less attention from researchers than one might expect, given the topic's importance. Nevertheless, surveying the limited literature in this field is still a challenge since it cuts across multiple areas: political science, public health, social policy, history, and more. Although not every study of alcohol policymaking can be discussed in detail in this section, a diverse range of key findings are reviewed to provide an overview of this essential topic.

One groundbreaking empirical study of alcohol policymaking, undertaken by Johnson and colleagues (2004), deserves investigation at some length. Johnson and colleagues examined the role of research in policy decisions about alcohol control at the federal level in the US primarily during the 1990s. Their findings were based upon numerous interviews conducted with members of executive and legislative branches of the US federal government, as well as with researchers, representatives from media outlets, and representatives from interest or pressure groups.

Johnson and colleagues found that research was more influential in the *early* stages of policymaking than in the *later* stages (p. 743). Specifically, research findings could help frame the agenda and designate a set of potential policy options; however, once bills had been proposed and began to be debated by policymakers, research was less influential than other concerns. These findings thus support the value of applying Kingdon's (2003) agenda-setting theory to alcohol policymaking, as it suggests that research can influence policy in specific ways during policymaking's early stages. These findings also echo a statement made in the World Health Organization Regional Office for Europe's (2009, p. 9) *Handbook for Action to Reduce Alcohol-Related Harm* that "Research appears to be most influential in setting a policy agenda and considering policy alternatives, less influential when amending draft laws and least influential in decision-making."

Johnson and colleagues also found that, when making policy decisions about alcohol, policymakers unsurprisingly placed greater value on other goals, such as boosting their prospects of getting re-elected, than on rigorously applying research evidence (pp. 743–4). Respondents in the study also admitted to deploying research for rhetorical purposes—e.g., to support their predetermined positions and to win favor with voters—rather than for informative purposes (pp. 744–5). Such findings match the claim made previously in this chapter that policymakers sometimes prefer "policy based evidence" and "look for evidence to support their claims" (Choi et al., 2005, p. 633).

A particularly difficult situation can arise when research evidence is complex and non-experts find it difficult to understand a policy's potential benefits. Johnson and colleagues noted the example of proposals advanced in the US in the 1990s that would increase national excise taxes on alcohol (pp. 747–8). However, it was not easy for experts to straightforwardly explain how such increases would directly decrease alcohol-related social harms, which made it difficult for such policies to obtain widespread support. Other policies for which this link was clearer, such as better enforcement of laws against alcohol-impaired driving, tended to be more popular with the public and were more likely to be adopted.

Another interesting examination of the interplay between evidence and alcohol policy was undertaken by Room (1991), who focused particularly on the US experience from the late nineteenth century to the 1980s. Room showed how key experts were influential in shaping approaches to alcohol use disorders, as well as public perceptions of individuals who suffered from such disorders (pp. 315–16); policymakers also drew upon social science and public health research during the latter part of this period to prove that alcohol misuse was a substantial problem (pp. 316–17). One compelling finding that emerged from Room's work was that experts *themselves* often profoundly disagreed about which alcohol policies were most likely to succeed, further complicating the relationship between research and policy.

Alcohol policymaking—and the role of evidence in the policy process—has of course not followed the same trajectory in every country, and such differences have encouraged the development of some alcohol policymaking studies with a distinctly national focus. For example, in his same historical overview, Room (1991, pp. 318–19) observed that, in the 1950s–1970s Finland demonstrated a particularly strong emphasis on using research evidence to shape alcohol policies—much more so than the US. Alavaikko and Österberg (2000) extended the study of Finland into the early 1990s, finding that the situation had changed sharply, with commercial interest groups exerting significant influence over alcohol policymaking, although after the passage of important alcohol-related legislation in 1994, their influence waned.

In Hungary, alcohol policymaking in the 1990s—a time of rapid political, economic, and social change that followed the fall of Communism—was explored by Varvasovszky and McKee (1998) in a series of interviews with key stakeholders who were involved in the alcohol policymaking process. They found that these stakeholders had no united vision of what the intended goals of alcohol policies were, and many important actors in the policy process were unaware of their potential power to foment policy change (p. 1824). Varvasovszky and McKee's findings are particularly interesting as they track alcohol policymaking during a time of political upheaval. The influence of historical changes on alcohol policymaking is an issue revisited in the next chapter.

Prohibition Movements and the Policy Process

Another informative area of research related to alcohol policymaking is the study of historical prohibition and temperance movements. Such movements attained great prominence in the US, the UK, Canada, Australia, and a number of other countries in the nineteenth and early twentieth centuries. Within ten years of the American Temperance Foundation's founding in 1826, 10 per cent of the country's population had joined its ranks (Morone, 2003, p. 284). In the UK, some temperance organizations—such as the children's group Band of Hope—achieved substantial influence during the Victorian and Edwardian eras (Barrow, 2003). The Australian temperance movement also gained influence during this period (Blainey, 2003) whilst in 1878 the Canada Temperance Act was passed, allowing municipalities to opt for local prohibitions on alcohol consumption ("The hemisphere", 1959).

Schrad (2010) has explored many of these groups' activities and efforts to influence policy, describing how temperance groups' cross-national communication ensured that ideas about limiting alcohol consumption spread across borders. This idea of cross-national communication among influential temperance leaders fits well with Dobbin and colleagues' (2007) first explanation of policy diffusion as driven by international networks of experts. According to Schrad (2010), World War I allowed prohibition advocates in a number of countries to link prohibition to patriotism (thus increasing the policy's appeal), although the specific policies adopted by the countries Schrad studied were diverse and influenced by each nation's particular political and governmental structure. This second finding echoes the emphasis in the broader policy diffusion literature about the tendency of policymakers to adapt policies to fit local conditions (Jones and Newburn, 2007, p. 7). Greenaway's (2003) work on historical alcohol policymaking within Britain adds the interesting finding that significant disagreement and in-fighting about alcohol policies occurred *within* or *among* temperance and alcohol abstinence organizations—as well as within governments and other stakeholder groups. The difficulty of establishing consensus even within a single stakeholder group likely impeded dramatic policy change. In Chapter 5, two lesser-known efforts to prohibit or sharply limit alcohol consumption—undertaken in Sri Lanka in 1904 and 1912 (Rogers, 1989) and in the Soviet Union in 1985 (Vågerö, 2011)—are explored in detail.

Policymaking and Illicit Drugs

Many interesting findings have emerged from studies examining policy decisions about illicit drugs, and given that alcohol is a drug, it is appropriate to consider prominent examples of the literature in this area.

Bennett and Holloway (2010), for example, who examined drug policymaking in the UK, found that although policy rhetoric often stressed the importance of learning from research evidence, difficulties in selecting, interpreting and reporting the results of evidence complicated this process. Such findings offer support for Head's (2008) assertion that the power of practical knowledge about policymaking should not be underestimated. Bennett and Holloway also reported that, in the realm of drug policymaking, policymakers and governments sometimes selectively deployed evidence to support their policy positions, and conveniently did not address studies that challenged their positions. This finding matches the theoretical assertion discussed earlier about policymakers' selective use of evidence (Choi et al., 2005, p. 633). Finally, Bennett and Holloway raised concerns that policymaking about drugs sometimes outpaced evidence-gathering, meaning that major decisions about policies were taken before a firm evidence base about those policies had developed. This finding mirrors Marmot's (2004) concerns about "policy based evidence" rather than "evidence based policy" that were outlined previously in this chapter.

A second revealing examination of evidence and drug policymaking was undertaken by Hughes and Stevens (2012), who focused on Portugal's 2001 policy change to decriminalize the possession of illicit drugs for personal use. Specifically, Hughes and Stevens highlighted "the misuse of evidence" and the "erroneous accounts" of the policy's effects that have marked some debates about the policy change (p. 110). Such errors in the way evidence is used and presented can have significant consequences, as they can "shift the debate on how reforms are spoken of" and change the public's beliefs about a policy (p. 110). Monaghan (2011, p. 42) has also explored the use of evidence in drug-related policymaking, arguing that "zero-sum" views that frame policies as either evidence-based or not evidence-based are misleading, as many gradations exist between these two extremes.

In another article, Stevens (2007) drew upon research into drug policymaking to posit an "evolutionary" theory about how certain ideas come to dominate policymaking. According to Stevens, the level of prominence that ideas gain is dependent upon how well they "fit the interests of powerful groups ... that can carry them into policy" (p. 28). In other words, the influence of ideas depends upon "the power of the carriers," or of the individuals who trumpet the ideas, "and the choices they make on which bits of evidence to pick up" (p. 28). Sadly, in Stevens' view, "the people whose interests are most directly harmed by these selective uses of evidence, being drug-using offenders and would-be immigrants and asylum seekers, are among the least powerful in these arguments," as they have the least ability to translate ideas into policy (p. 30). This emphasis on power dynamics echoes, in a more cynical fashion, Weiss' (1983) idea that competing interests and power imbalances shape the policymaking process.

The Alcohol Industry

Weiss' idea of competing interests also connects to another prominent theme in the alcohol policymaking literature: the involvement of the alcohol industry in shaping policy. Greenfield, Johnson, and Giesbrecht (2004) conducted interviews with public health advocates operating at the national level in the US; such advocates often expressed the belief that the alcohol industry exerted a strong influence over alcohol policymaking given its extensive campaign donations and lobbying efforts. These beliefs seem borne out by the fact that, in the late 1990s, according to Greenfield and colleagues, the heads of two major alcohol industry lobbying groups were former members of Congress.

The alcohol industry's involvement in policymaking is not unique to the US. Stevens (2007, p. 30), for example, has similarly posited that the Portman Group, an organization funded by the alcohol industry, may have influenced the use of evidence in the UK government's 2004 alcohol strategy. Bakke and Endal's (2010) research, discussed previously in this chapter, also highlighted the alcohol industry's involvement in alcohol policymaking in several sub-Saharan African countries.

Of course the alcohol industry does not necessarily dominate alcohol policymaking to the exclusion of all other interest groups. Greenfield and colleagues' (2004) interviews, for example, reveal that public health advocates also typically expressed a firm belief that activist organizations could gain prominence in alcohol policymaking by mobilizing public support and spearheading campaigns to encourage citizens to contact their governmental representatives.

Additionally, it is important to recognize that the alcohol industry is not the only interest group with a clear economic stake in many alcohol policy decisions. The resources available to alcohol researchers, treatment specialists, public health advocates, and others are also often affected by alcohol policy decisions, and this relationship should not be overlooked. More than 15 years ago Hanson (1995, p. 30) cautioned that estimates of the proportion of Americans who engage in harmful drinking practices could be "inflated by a diversity of entrepreneurs who have a vested interest in exaggerating the extent of drinking problems." Hanson's provocative argument highlights the importance of recognizing that an entire industry—and many thousands of jobs—have developed to minimize and treat alcohol's social harms. Like the alcohol retail industry, this industry of remediation is, to a degree, economically dependent on alcohol policies.

Other Issues

In addition to policymaking and policy diffusion, policy *implementation* is also a critical step in the alcohol policy process. Policy implementation is "the process of putting policy into action" and "the realization of a policy decision" (Sapru, 2010, p. 221). Sidlow and Henschen's (2009, p. 341) definition of policymaking, described at the beginning of this chapter, includes "implementing a policy" as a key component of policymaking. As early as 1989, Mosher and Jernigan stressed the importance of implementation and expressed concern that the alcohol industry could hinder the implementation of evidence-based policies. Similarly, more than two decades ago Beauvais (1992) published an article titled "The Need for Community Consensus as a Condition of Policy Implementation in the Reduction of Alcohol Abuse on Indian Reservations," which explored the unique considerations that need to be taken into account when implementing alcohol policies in Native American reservations. However despite these and some other exceptions, implementation has received much less attention than other aspects of alcohol policymaking (Wagenaar and Toomey, 2000, p. 687).

In addition to policy implementation, a related issue that deserves mention here is policy *enforcement*. Many policies that aim to reduce alcohol's social harms have little or no effect if they are not enforced. Pechansky and Chandran (2012), for example, have noted that although some countries in Latin America and South America have laws limiting drivers' BAC to 0.05 g/dl—a limit stricter than that in place in the US—many of these countries still have very high levels of alcohol-related traffic crashes. According to Pechansky and Chandran, such high levels of crashes are due in part to a dearth of resources for enforcement in these countries. More broadly, measuring the extent to which alcohol policies are enforced in various countries is critical in order to make meaningful cross-national comparisons of alcohol policy regimes. As Ritter (2007) and Brand and colleagues (2007) have observed, one useful metric for comparing countries' alcohol policies *does not* take into account enforcement, as information on enforcement around the world can be difficult to obtain. Despite the fundamental importance of enforcement, like implementation, it has also traditionally received less attention from researchers than other topics related to alcohol policymaking (Wagenaar and Toomey, 2000, p. 687).

Conclusion

Perhaps the most striking overall conclusion that can be drawn from this review is the incredible *variety* of perspectives that scholars have developed to explain policymaking and to explore evidence's impact. The answer to the question which introduced this chapter—"what factors influence the alcohol policymaking process?"—can thus be seen to be multifaceted. From Lasswell's (1951) optimism for empirical research's potential for solving social problems, to Stevens' (2007) evolutionary theory of drug policymaking, a diverse range of theories and studies have been advanced. Many of these perspectives could not be more different from each other. The questions of which of these perspectives offers the *most* insight into alcohol policymaking, and whether the myriad ideas advanced in this chapter hold any explanatory value in the area of alcohol policymaking, are probed through the case studies presented throughout the rest of this book.

Finally, it is necessary to identify a major potential limitation of many of the theories outlined here—namely, the question of their *international* applicability. Although some findings from sub-Saharan Africa and South America were briefly mentioned in this chapter, the majority of the research that has been conducted on alcohol policymaking and the role of evidence has focused on western, developed countries. Is policy making in *non*-western, and less developed countries also conducted in an incremental fashion (Lindblom, 1959; 1979)? Does policy learning also drive policy diffusion in such settings (Dobbin et al., 2007)? The next chapter explores these kinds of questions in detail, and examines the wider issue of how both globalization and countries' specific characteristics shape alcohol policymaking.

Chapter 4
History, Culture, Context, and Transformation

"A gin-sodden mother is oblivious to her child's fall. Addiction to spirits leads to negligence, poverty and death." This is how the British Museum's website describes *Gin Lane*, a 1751 print by the English artist William Hogarth. In exacting detail, *Gin Lane* (shown in Figure 4.1 on the following page) depicts gin as the bringer of chaos, devastation, violence, and tragedy to London's streets. The print is a fictionalized, yet disturbing, portrayal of a real historical case study—the 1720s–1750s English "gin craze"—which offers lessons for contemporary debates about alcohol control.

During this period, the consumption of gin in England rose sharply, and many observers believed this increase was associated with an epidemic of the social harms depicted in Hogarth's print (McIntosh, 2003; Phillips, 2003). Gin was first developed in Holland in the mid seventeenth century and by the early eighteenth century had been introduced to Britain by soldiers returning from the Continent (Rodin, 1981, p. 1237). In 1689 Parliament made a policy change which allowed anyone to open a distillery, as long as they could pay the required fee (Abel, 2001, p. 401). To serve the interests of major landowners—whose land produced the wheat from which gin was fermented—taxes on gin were initially kept at a low level (Warren and Bast, 1988, p. 638). Thus gin gained a crucial tax advantage over ale and beer (Rodin, 1981, p. 1237).

According to official figures analyzed by Abel (2001, p. 401), gin consumption more than tripled between 1714 and 1751, from 2 to over 7 million gallons per year, while consumption of beer approximately held steady. Per capita consumption of gin likely peaked in 1743 at 2.2 gallons per year (Warner, 2002, p. 3). However, as Phillips (2003, p. 265) has noted, accounting for illicit gin and the demographics of consumption could boost these figures yet higher, suggesting that, in London "adult men must have had easy access to up to ten gallons of spirits a year, about a modern bottle per weak." As the "gin craze" escalated, the resultant social problems associated with this increase in alcohol consumption received significant public attention (Phillips, 2003; Porter, 1985). Medical experts in Georgian England regularly asserted that alcohol was a driver of poor health, and thus discouraged excessive alcohol consumption (Porter, 1985). Reformers such as Henry Fielding, a magistrate in Westminster, linked the consumption of gin to infant mortality, crime, and other social harms (Dillon, 2002).

Warner (1994b) has argued that the public outcry was, in part, due to the changes in alcohol consumption patterns that gin prompted. Gin's relatively

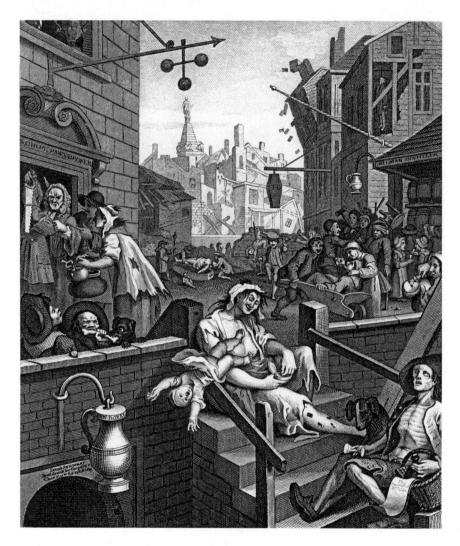

Figure 4.1   *Gin Lane* (1751), print by William Hogarth

low cost in comparison to other alcoholic drinks meant that poorer people could consume large quantities. According to Warner, gin was also sold on the streets and in other areas that were not traditional sites of alcohol retail sales, prompting further concern. In addition, women participated more widely in the gin trade than they had in the trade for other kinds of alcohol, both as sellers of gin and possibly also as consumers (particularly since sweetened gin was considered "a woman's drink") (Phillips, 2003, p. 265). Warner (1994b) has posited that this subversion of gender norms may have heightened concern about gin.

During the gin craze, gin was often negatively contrasted with beer and ale (Warner, 1995a). Indeed, Hogarth also issued a second print titled *Beer Street* in 1751. This work depicts the orderly contentment that results from the traditional consumption of English ale—a scene that stands in sharp contrast to the dissolution portrayed in *Gin Lane* (The British Museum, n.d.). At the time that Hogarth produced his prints, ale had long been consumed in England whilst gin—as described above—was a new, foreign beverage (Rodin, 1981). This "foreignness" likely also contributed to the concern that arose about the gin craze. Interestingly, Yeomans (2009) has observed that the reaction to the gin craze differed from later, nineteenth-century British temperance movements as reformers did not typically view alcohol itself as the problem—rather, the harms resulting from excessive consumption were the focus of reformers' concern. One can see this nuance clearly in *Beer Street*, which emphasizes the happy consequences of moderate consumption.

In an attempt to reduce gin's social harms, legislation was adopted in 1735 which instituted taxes and license charges on gin retailers; the act specifically cited concern about the social harms arising from excessive gin consumption (as quoted in Haslam, 1996, p. 123). Yet the act was so unpopular and difficult to enforce that it was repealed in 1743 following a series of impassioned parliamentary debates (Haslam, 1996). In these debates some politicians emphasized the terrible human costs of excessive gin consumption, while others argued that so many individuals were involved in the gin trade that regulations were futile; in language reminiscent of contemporary debates the Bishop of Sarum pleaded in the House of Lords that politicians remember "the children, my lords" who could be affected by gin's harms (as quoted in Lees, 1864, p. 66).

Seven years after the act's repeal, the House of Commons continued to receive numerous pleas for action to be taken regarding the gin craze; one such petition from the Lord Mayor of London focused on gin's health consequences and its associations with violence. Specifically, the Lord Mayor wrote that "the common and habitual use of spirituous liquors by the lower ranks of people ... inflames them with rage and barbarity, and occasions frequent robberies and murders in the streets of the Metropolis" (as quoted in Lees, 1864, p. 67). The following year, 1751, Hogarth released *Gin Lane* as part of a large, concerted campaign to reduce the consumption of gin (British Museum, n.d.). According to Hogarth, copies of *Gin Lane* were published "in the cheapest Manner possible" to encourage their wide distribution, although the print's price of one shilling would still have been out of reach for many of the poor (as quoted in Paulson, 1993, p. 26). The wider campaign that *Gin Lane* was part of ultimately achieved success, for later in 1751 the Tippling Act was passed, which restricted the sale of gin from shops selling everyday household necessities and endeavored to limit the manufacture and sale of gin to larger retail outlets (British Museum, n.d.; Emmons, 2000, pp. 159–60). Harsh sentences—including imprisonment in severe cases—were specified for those who disobeyed the Tippling Act (Abel, 2001, p. 401).

In the years immediately following the act's passage the price of gin increased sharply and consumption decreased (Emmons, 2000); however, some observers have questioned whether the act was the sole or primary cause of the abatement in the gin craze (Phillips, 2003, p. 265). Although gin consumption fell dramatically, beer consumption slightly rose in the years following the Act's adoption (Abel, 2001, p. 401). Interestingly, even though, as Hogarth's *Beer Street* print reveals, beer (and, more specifically, ale) was often viewed as a less dangerous alternative to gin, the rise in beer consumption that followed the Tippling Act *itself* prompted concern, and legislation was passed in 1753 making it more difficult to gain a license to sell ale (Lees, 1864, p. 69).

The gin craze and the introduction of the Tippling Act constitute one of the best-known examples of how alcohol's social harms can prompt dramatic policy changes. Indeed, these events set an important precedent, promoting a greater role for governments in addressing social problems such as alcohol misuse (Critcher, 2011; Davison, 1992). They also reveal how debates about alcohol use can be intertwined with larger social issues, such as class divisions and urbanization (Warner, 2002). In more recent times, the gin craze and the Tippling Act have been analyzed to see what specific lessons they might offer for contemporary efforts to tackle alcohol's social harms (e.g., Borsay, 2007; Thompson, 2012b; Warner, 1994b). Warner (1994b), for example, has explored the similarities between the gin craze and the US crack cocaine epidemic of the 1980s and early 1990s, noting that both phenomena featured a preoccupation with poor, urban mothers. In the American crack epidemic, such concern was evident in media attention given to "crack babies"—children born to drug-using mothers—while in the gin craze such concern is depicted by Hogarth's portrayal of a gin-using mother's ignorance of her falling child.

Ultimately, the reaction to the gin craze illustrates that public and governmental concerns about alcohol's social harms have a long history. These concerns can be shaped by changes in drinking patterns, as well as by cultural attitudes—such as, in this case, attitudes about women's societal roles—and by political and economic factors. Such concerns can, in turn, be mobilized by reformers to instigate policy change. The gin craze is also important because it offers an example of the ways in which historical experiences—or the collective memories and understandings of such experiences—can influence later alcohol policymaking. Perhaps in part because of Hogarth's memorable works, this historical phenomenon has had a lasting effect on British culture and attitudes to alcohol. Indeed, even a 2010 article published in *The Telegraph* about the contemporary problem of binge drinking referenced "Hogarth's Gin Lane" (Humphrys, 2010). As the British Museum's official description of Hogarth's print explains: "The horrors of *Gin Lane* provided imagery for propaganda against alcohol for another hundred years." The fact that the gin craze is still referenced in contemporary debates illustrates the potency of history—or, at least, society's collective interpretation of such history.

Beyond the Gin Craze

In addition to the gin craze, other historical phenomena have also cast long shadows over British alcohol policymaking. For example, the British temperance movement that gained prominence in the nineteenth century "had a decisive impact on the way alcohol is viewed in Britain," as it cast alcohol's negative impacts as important social and political issues (Yeomans, 2009, p. 3.1). Similarly, in the US the Prohibition Era of the early twentieth century has left a lasting legacy. Even today Prohibition's perceived failures are often cited in debates about restricting alcohol's availability, as seen in relation to the Oglala Sioux Tribe's policy of prohibiting alcohol at the Pine Ridge Reservation, discussed in Chapter 1. Specifically, in an article responding to this case for the *Huffington Post*, a representative of the Drug Policy Alliance referenced the problems of the Prohibition Era (Newman, 2012). The fact that Prohibition's lack of success was mentioned in a publication aimed at a popular audience without any further explanation or context shows the continuing currency of this event in American debates.

In addition to historical events, historical drinking patterns and attitudes to alcohol also influence contemporary discourse. Engs (1995), for example, has explored how historical factors may have impacted the development of different drinking patterns across Europe, resulting in different drinking cultures that still affect alcohol consumption patterns today. Specifically, Engs has examined suggestions that, historically, unpredictable weather or changing trade patterns made alcohol periodically scarce in northern Europe in previous centuries; this scarcity contrasted sharply with the more consistent availability of alcohol (and, in particular, wine) in many parts of southern Europe. According to Engs, the fluctuating availability of alcohol in northern Europe may have encouraged the development of more binge-oriented drinking patterns, while the more consistent availability of alcohol in southern Europe may have encouraged the development of more moderate drinking patterns. Österberg and Karlsson (2002, p. 18) have also noted that, in many parts of southern Europe, strict cultural norms often specify when, and how much, can be consumed. These cultural norms explain why little formal regulation of alcohol retail sales was in place in much of this region several decades ago. In contrast, much of northern Europe—where cultural norms governing alcohol have not been as restrictive—traditionally has seen much stronger formal regulation governing alcohol. The role of culture in influencing drinking patterns is explored in more detail in the next section.

The influence of history can be seen far beyond Europe as well. Prior to contact with Europeans, Native Americans in the southwest US, Mexico, Central America, and Amazon regions typically only consumed alcohol during religious rites (Hernandez-Avila and Kranzler, 2011, p. 139), yet today, as stated in Chapter 2, Native Americans now have the highest alcohol-related mortality rates of any ethnic group in the US (McFarland et al., 2006; National Institute on Alcohol Abuse and Alcoholism, 2007). As Frank, Moore, and Ames (2000) have argued, such contemporary alcohol consumption patterns among Native Americans can only be understood by examining the major historical influence of European conquest, colonization, and colonialism.

The influence of history can also be detected in Mexico, where, based upon anthropological research on fiestas in one local community, Pérez (2000, p. 365) concluded that: "The perpetuation of binge drinking and violence are part of a historic cycle of male dominance that dates back to the introduction of alcohol distillation during colonization by the Spaniards in the 16th century." Such findings reveal how historical and cultural factors can intersect and still affect contemporary attitudes toward alcohol.

One final example that deserves mention is that of South Africa, where some illegal alcohol outlets, known as shebeens, played a role in helping to foment organized resistance to apartheid from the 1950s onward (Parry, 2005, p. 426). The shebeens provided a place where black South Africans could socialize "beyond the scrutiny of the state" and additionally "helped to sustain a vibrant subculture that emerged in the shadow of the establishment of apartheid" (Ambler, 2003, p. 13). This idea that alcohol outlets can serve not only a social function, but also a transformative political purpose, resonates in studies beyond South Africa. According to Scott (1990, p. 121), for example, throughout centuries of European history, "the alehouse, the pub, the tavern, the inn, the cabaret … were seen by secular authorities and by the church as places of subversion. Here subordinate classes met offstage and off-duty in an atmosphere of freedom encouraged by alcohol." Thompson (1999, p. 19) has similarly written of the importance of taverns in shaping the political culture in Philadelphia, where, "in the first two-thirds of the eighteenth century" such premises provided places of assembly where "men from different ranks and ethnicities discussed politics in an atmosphere remarkably free from deference". A similar phenomenon was present in the early 1960s in Ghana, where "drinking bars became active places of political resistance" to the ruling party, and helped foment public feelings before a general strike in 1961 (Akyeampong, 1996, p. 147).

Just as drinking can be connected to greater social and political changes, attempts to control drinking can also have political implications as well. Conroy (1995, p. 8), for example, has described how "the regulations of taverns" in Puritan-era New England was "part of the maintenance of a deferential political system." The proliferation of alehouses in seventeenth-century England similarly worried political and social elites, given, as previously mentioned, these premises' "potential as disruptive influences" to the social and political fabric (Smyth, 2004, p. xx; Clark, 1983). Such historical examples suggest that, in order to fully analyze drinking practices as well as alcohol policies themselves, one must situate such practices and policies within their proper historical contexts, probing whether they reflect relevant political and societal power dynamics. The connection between alcohol policies and wider political and social themes is revisited later in several of this book's case studies.

Cultural and Social Contexts

Some of the most influential insights into the relationship between alcohol and culture were revealed by the American anthropologist Dwight B. Heath in a 1958 academic paper about the drinking patterns of the Camba people in Bolivia. Heath reported that although the Camba traditionally drank large amounts of very strong alcohol at their many festive events, the social harms traditionally associated with excessive alcohol consumption—such as violence, disorder, or alcoholism—did not typically afflict their society. Such findings imply that cultural and even situational factors can impact whether, and to what extent, disorder and even violence accompany excessive alcohol consumption. Malcolm Gladwell described Heath's research in a 2010 article in *The New Yorker*. In the article, Gladwell emphasized the role of cultural factors in mediating reactions to alcohol—including the emergence of social harms—writing that: "There is something about the cultural dimension of social problems that eludes us. When confronted with the rowdy youth in the bar, we are happy to raise his drinking age, to tax his beer … But we are reluctant to provide him with a positive and constructive example of how to drink" (p. 76).

Providing "a positive and constructive example of how to drink" is commonly said to be a feature of some drinking cultures, such as those of France and Italy. Indeed, as early as Victorian times, the "French" or "continental" style of drinking was advocated as a model that British drinkers should follow to reduce alcohol's social harms (Nicholls, 2012). However, in more recent years, the belief that French drinking patterns might serve as a positive model has been challenged by reports that binge drinking is on the rise in France—and in particular that the traditional French taboo against public drunkenness is being increasingly broken by students (Doust, 2007).

In addition to *international* differences in culture and attitudes to alcohol, scholars have also identified significant *intra-national* differences that are worth exploring. For example, a British Medical Association (2008) report about UK drinking patterns revealed that 90 percent of individuals of Pakistani and Bangladeshi origin did not drink alcohol, compared with almost half of individuals of African or Caribbean origin, and with just 9 percent of individuals of white British origin. These dramatic differences suggest that cultural factors—such as high rates of adherence to Islam among those of Pakistani and Bangladeshi origin—can indeed influence drinking patterns. The relationship between religious affiliations and attitudes or policies toward alcohol has received much attention from researchers (Holt et al., 2006). The importance of this relationship is underlined by Room and colleagues' (2005, p. 519) observation that "every major world religion has at least some strands that counsel abstinence from alcohol beverages." One example of this relationship can be identified in the US state of Utah where the Mormon Church—which disapproves of alcohol consumption—is headquartered. Utah has traditionally maintained much more restrictive policies governing alcohol sales than many other US states, and despite a liberalization of such restrictions in 2009, as of this writing, "happy hours" are still banned and restaurant patrons who order alcohol must also order food (Cooper, 2011).

Of course it must always be remembered that the influence of religion and other cultural factors is not constant; within religious denominations and other subsections of society, individuals hold different views, and these views can change over time. In line with this idea, Brugha and Varvasovszky (2000) have noted that the stakeholders involved in policymaking do not represent monolithic, unchanging interests; instead, they are also affected by social, political, historical, and economic forces. This observation adds further complexity to Weiss' (1983) idea—outlined in the previous chapter—that competing interests can drive policymaking. It is important to recognize that such interests can also change over time, and can be shaped by contexts and evolving political and economic circumstances.

At the heart of all of the theories and observations discussed here is a Durkheimian emphasis on social factors that affect individual behaviors—including individual reactions to alcohol. As Gladwell (2010, p. 76) has posited: "Culture is a more powerful tool in dealing with drinking than medicine, economics, or the law." Of course, alcohol intoxication itself is a biological state which involves biochemical and mechanical changes in a drinker's body; drunkenness, however, and the behaviors that an intoxicated person displays are socially-conditioned (Stockley and Saunders, 2010).

More broadly, psychologists in recent years have paid increasing attention to how social contexts can shape behavior (Matsumoto, 2007), and understanding how drinking contexts shape drinking practices is also fundamental. Alcohol outlets—such as community pubs or saloons—are acknowledged as serving as a "third place," separate from home and work, where people can socialize in a relatively safe environment (Oldenburg, 1997; 2001). The social importance of alcohol outlets has also been examined by Graham (2005, p. 48) who remarked in one historical study of public drinking that "if intoxication and addiction were the sole reasons for consuming alcohol, there would be little reason for the existence of public houses," since consuming alcohol in private can satisfy both of these goals. The work of anthropologists has helped illuminate the effects of context, culture, and location on drinking and alcohol-related social behaviors (see, e.g., Douglas, 1987). Indeed, as Heath (1987, p. 16) wrote more than 25 years ago about the contributions of anthropological perspectives on drinking: "Even practitioners of the so-called 'hard sciences' acknowledge that social and cultural factors must be taken into account, together with physiological and psychological factors, when one attempts to understand the interaction of alcohol and behavior." Both cultural and individual factors can influence the behaviors—and social harms—that result from alcohol consumption.

This idea is evidenced in the literature on alcohol "expectancies"—or people's expectations about alcohol's effects (Arriola et al., 2009; Christiansen, Goldman, and Inn, 1982). Studies of alcohol expectancies explore the social, psychological, and other effects that people sometimes experience when they *think* they are drinking alcohol, but in reality are merely consuming a placebo (Testa et al., 2006). The existence of such expectancies—i.e., the fact that some individuals can believe they are experiencing social and psychological effects when they are consuming nonalcoholic placebo beverages—underlines the importance of context, culture, and socialization in influencing drinking behaviors and reactions to alcohol consumption.

Although ideas about the effects of context and culture on drinking pervade the academic literature, discussing such effects in a policy context can be surprisingly controversial. In October 2011, a commentator named Kate Fox wrote the following in an editorial on the BBC News website: "Clearly, we Brits do have a bit of a problem with alcohol, but why? The problem is that we Brits believe that alcohol ... causes us to shed our inhibitions and become aggressive, promiscuous, disorderly and even violent. But we are wrong." Instead, Fox argued that "the effects of alcohol on behavior are determined by cultural rules and norms, not by the chemical actions of ethanol." She claimed that the best way to reduce alcohol's harmful impact on British society would be to encourage personal responsibility and change the public's expectations about alcohol use. According to Fox, if people believed that alcohol was *not* necessarily associated with inhibition shedding, they would be less likely to shed their inhibitions when drunk. Fox asserted that removing alcohol's mystical aura and making consumption seem pedestrian would reduce its social harms. Fox's argument deeply divided website readers, however. Her editorial attracted an astounding number of comments—over 1,000 within 24 hours of posting.

Yet Fox's more general point that reshaping public beliefs about drinking might reduce alcohol's social harms has also been advanced by other commentators. For example, de Castella (2012) has described concerns that exaggerated beliefs about the prevalence of excessive drinking among one's peers or in society at large might actually *encourage* individuals to drink too much. Therefore, showing that excessive drinking is less common than some believe might result in a decrease in excessive consumption and its related harms.

Globalization and Macro Changes

It is important to recognize that the cross-national differences in drinking cultures discussed in the previous section are themselves subject to historical political and economic forces. Macro-level trends, such as increasing globalization, are impacting drinking patterns. To see this clearly, it is useful to focus on the example of Europe. As described earlier, historical scholarship has examined the development of more binge-oriented drinking patterns in parts of northern Europe and more moderate drinking patterns in parts of southern Europe (Engs, 1995). Yet today differences in drinking cultures between northern and southern Europeans seem to be narrowing and "converging"—particularly among young people (Beccaria and White, 2012, p. 36). This departure from the traditional drinking patterns of the past can be traced in part to the forces of globalization (Rehm et al., 2003, p. 154).

Such globalizing forces have not only encouraged the convergence of drinking patterns, but have also, alongside technological change and greater communications, facilitated the cross-national *diffusion* of alcohol policies themselves. Theories of policy diffusion were explored in detail in the previous chapter; such theories posit that networks of international experts, coercion by international organizations, and policy learning can all promote the spread of policies across borders (Dobbin et al., 2007). One example of policy diffusion in the alcohol sphere can be found, once again, in Europe. Within the EU, countries have, in recent times, increasingly turned away from import controls that limit alcohol's availability, in part due to the EU's emphasis on free trade across European borders (Ahlström et al., 2004; Bentzen and Smith, 2004; National Institute for Health and Welfare, 2012). The fact that EU priorities have influenced European countries' choices about alcohol policies offers some support for Dobbin and colleagues' (2007) ideas, discussed in the previous chapter, that supranational organizations can play a key role in policy diffusion by encouraging countries to adopt particular policies.

Investigating this example further, it is important to note that, although in previous decades the EU's priority on the issue of alcohol was to break down trade barriers among countries and to ensure alcohol was properly taxed, from the 1990s onward the promotion of public health has become increasingly significant as well (Alavaikko and Österberg, 2000; National Institute for Health and Welfare, 2012; Tigerstedt, 1990). Since 1999, within the European Commission, the Directorate-General for Health and Consumer Protection (DG SANCO) has overseen issues related to alcohol and health (Örnberg, 2013). In 2006, the Commission released its *Strategy to Support Member States in Reducing Alcohol-Related Harm*— considered the first official EU "alcohol strategy" (National Institute for Health and Welfare, 2012). The strategy's objectives include reducing underage drinking and prenatal exposure to alcohol, decreasing alcohol-impaired driving through tough and well-enforced blood-alcohol limits, and compiling more accurate data on the extent of harmful drinking in Europe (*European strategy* ..., 2011). The Nordic countries played a key role in the design and eventual adoption of the alcohol strategy (National Institute for Health and Welfare, 2012)—an involvement which is not surprising, given these countries' traditional emphasis on formal (rather than informal) strategies to reduce alcohol's social harms. In addition to the formal European strategy, international groups such as the Alcohol Policy Network in Europe (2012) have also emerged in recent years to share knowledge about best practices and promote policymaking that regulates alcohol. This internationalization of knowledge about preventing alcohol's social harms reflects the international emphasis of the WHO's (2010) Global Strategy on alcohol.

Of course, it is essential not to overstate the convergence in European alcohol policies. Despite these trends, countries' policies are not identical. For example, taxes remain greatest in the UK, Ireland, and the Nordic countries, and are typically lower in wine-producing countries (Babor, 2004, p. 41). As discussed in the previous chapter, such differences mean that one cannot expect that a policy that developed in one culture or country can simply be transferred unchanged to another culture or country, despite the power of globalization and other convergence-promoting forces.

Developed and Developing Countries

Related to this theme is the question—addressed in the concluding section of the previous chapter—of whether policies that have been found to be successful in developed countries could also work in developing countries. The fact that much previous research on alcohol policymaking has focused on western, developed countries means that important gaps exist in experts' knowledge about "what works" in the developing world.

Developing countries are not immune from the globalizing forces that have also affected policymaking in developed countries. Indeed, the previous chapter outlined Bakke and Endal's (2010) research about the multinational alcohol industry's attempts to influence policy in four sub-Saharan African countries. Bakke and Endal discovered that the alcohol industry encouraged the adoption of similar policies in all four of these countries, illustrating the alcohol industry's influence in the developing world—and also suggesting that external foreign businesses can sometimes work to ensure their economic interests take precedence over other concerns in the alcohol policy process. Exploring a related issue, Caetano and Laranjeira (2006, p. 150) have highlighted the efforts of multinational alcohol conglomerates to buy up parts of the local alcohol industry in developing countries—a move that can further cement such conglomerates' power. These points underline the importance of exploring the potential influence of the alcohol industry over policymaking in developed countries. In this aspect, alcohol policymaking in developing countries is similar to that in developed countries, where—as explored in detail in the previous chapter—the alcohol industry also can exert significant influence (Greenfield, Johnson, and Giesbrecht, 2004; Stevens, 2007).

A more comprehensive portrait of alcohol policymaking in developing countries is offered in Thamarangsi's (2008) study of Thailand between 1997 and 2006. During this period, Thai alcohol policy became broader and more focused on promoting public health. In addition, according to Thamarangsi, during these years the government placed increasing emphasis on tackling alcohol's social harms and solving problems related to misuse—although issues of promoting commerce and economic growth remained important. Thamarangsi's research indicates that, in general, the development of alcohol policies received more attention in Thailand during this period than their implementation or follow-up; in particular, a lack of resources and problems with management sometimes impeded these latter two processes. Finally, and perhaps most interestingly, Thamarangsi (2008, p. i) found that "Incrementalism characterised Thai alcohol policy formulation; existing policy or the policy precursor was very important to the decisions made." In other words,

Thailand's experiences seem to offer support for Lindblom's (1959; 1979) thesis, explored in detail in the previous chapter, that policymaking typically consists of small, incremental changes rather than dramatic changes, with policymakers often adopting new policies that are often quite similar to the policies already in place.

Another issue to address on the theme of alcohol policymaking in developed and developing countries is the idea that increasing wealth is sometimes associated with increasing alcohol use. As mentioned in Chapter 2, total global consumption of alcohol—and the social harms related to consumption—will likely increase in future years, as economic growth in countries like India and China creates more demand (Harrell, 2009; Rehm, Patra, et al., 2006; Rehm et al., 2009). Consuming alcohol costs money; as developing countries' economies strengthen, their citizens have more resources available to purchase alcohol. Even within developed countries, money seems to be associated with alcohol consumption. For example, a British report found that employed individuals were more likely to consume alcohol frequently than those without jobs—suggesting that the more mundane issue of having enough money to purchase alcohol can also impact drinking habits (British Medical Association, 2008). Ultimately these examples illustrate that, in addition to macro-level political, historical, and cultural factors, individual economic factors might also influence patterns of alcohol use.

Public Opinion

A final theme related to culture that is essential to examine in this chapter is public opinion, and its role in encouraging the adoption of alcohol policies. The importance of public support can be seen in the work of Johnson and colleagues' (2004, pp. 747–8), who have described how proposals to increase national excise taxes on alcohol in the US in the 1990s were not adopted in part because of the lack of public support. The complexities of public opinion have been further explored by Österberg (2007) in an analysis of Finnish alcohol policies. Österberg found that public support for greater alcohol restrictions in Finland decreased in the 1960s. However, in the 1970s, as alcohol-related social harms appeared to be on the increase, public support for restrictions *increased*. In the 1980s, although alcohol consumption and related social harms continued to rise, public support for restrictions fell again. These complex findings indicate that the relationship between alcohol-related harm and public opinion about alcohol restrictions is not always straightforward or constant. Indeed, the finding that public opinion about alcohol policies can change over time has been echoed in the work of Giesbrecht and colleagues (2007), which explored Canadian public opinion data about alcohol control policies in 1989, 1994, and 2004. Giesbrecht and colleagues found that support for restrictive policies *declined* over time, demonstrating once again that opinion can vary in response to evolving patterns of alcohol use or other major changes in society.

The influence of public opinion over alcohol policymaking can sharply increase when such opinion is mobilized by influential organized groups. Johnson and colleagues (2004) have posited that Mothers Against Drunk Driving (MADD), a pressure group in the US, did much to increase awareness about the harms of alcohol-impaired driving and encourage policy change (Treuthart, 2005, pp. 108–9; Voas and Fell, 2010). The example of early-twentieth-century American Prohibition, a dramatic policy change whose adoption was encouraged by organized temperance groups (Schrad, 2010), further highlights the potential of such groups to harness the public sentiment of some sectors in society, and take action. This idea is explored in greater detail in Chapter 7.

Conclusion

One cannot fully understand societies' patterns of alcohol consumption without examining the cultural, historical, political, economic, and other factors that can shape such patterns. These factors can also affect attitudes to alcohol and beliefs about alcohol policymaking, thereby potentially impacting the policies countries adopt to combat alcohol's social harms as well. This chapter's findings underline the importance of considering anthropological work—such as Heath's (1958; 1987) landmark research—when exploring drinking patterns and the cultural role of alcohol. In order to design effective and publicly-supported alcohol policies, such findings need to be a key component of the public health approach to alcohol policy.

Indeed, one can see how such factors affected the class- and gender-based aspects of the reaction to the eighteenth-century British "gin craze" discussed at the beginning of this chapter. This point about the importance of cultural, historical, political, and economic factors has one further implication—it means that alcohol policies cannot always be straightforwardly transferred across countries. Policies that have produced positive results in one historical or cultural context are not guaranteed to be effective elsewhere, as countries have different cultures and political systems—in addition to varying levels of alcohol abuse and unique prevention needs. Thus, although societies can learn from other societies' experiences, it is important to recognize that policies to control alcohol abuse must often be adapted to fit local contexts. To offer one example of this phenomenon, Babor and Caetano (2005) have described how several Latin American countries have adopted a wide range of tailored prevention strategies to address local priorities related to alcohol's social harms.

When adapting alcohol policies to fit local contexts, it is important to take into account practical considerations. One such practical consideration, as König and Segura (2011) have detailed, is the level of *infrastructure* present within a society. Such infrastructure is comprised of the resources, personnel, and organizations available within a country to design and implement effective public health practices. Although a proposed policy may be evidence-based, if a country lacks the infrastructure to implement it, such a policy is unlikely to succeed. Tailoring policies to account for countries' levels of infrastructure could thus likely facilitate the diffusion of alcohol policies across borders.

Of course, it is important not to overstate the influence of culture and the environment, or to mistakenly attribute biologically-caused results to cultural and environmental factors. Chrzan (2011, p. 122), for example, has expressed concern that some cross-cultural studies of drinking are guilty of "embracing too enthusiastically the socially constitutive aspects of alcohol use." On the other hand, according to Chrzan, other studies can be equally guilty of promoting a "lack of cultural contextualization" (p. 122). The case studies presented in the book's remaining chapters endeavor to achieve this balance between appreciating the effects of culture and context without overstating their influence.

Chapter 5
Key Lessons from Prohibition Policies: Beyond the 1920s

The story of American Prohibition—and the speakeasies, bathtub-gin syndicates, and gangsterism it gave rise to—is well-known.[1] However, many other examples of policy moves to prohibit—or nearly prohibit—alcohol also deserve attention. For example, Chapter 1 highlighted the Oglala Sioux Nation's efforts to enforce prohibition on the Pine Ridge Reservation in South Dakota. This chapter explores two other twentieth-century efforts to prohibit or sharply reduce alcohol consumption: the first in the Soviet Union in the 1980s, and the second in Sri Lanka in the early twentieth century. These two very different case studies were selected to explore the diversity of factors that can affect efforts to influence alcohol policy. Through these case studies, the explanatory value of the policymaking theories discussed in Chapter 3 and the contextual factors outlined in Chapter 4 can be assessed.

In one sense, the policies described in both of these case studies were "failures". The Soviet Union's campaign did not produce long-lasting declines in consumption and sadly resulted in numerous deaths from the underground consumption of homemade alcoholic beverages (Nemtsov, 2011; "Prohibition, Soviet style", 1990). The campaign in Sri Lanka gained considerable political influence, but, against the backdrop of colonial rule, did not succeed in fomenting national restrictions on alcohol (Bond, 1988; Rogers, 1989). Yet even these policy "failures" constitute valuable opportunities for learning about the factors that can facilitate or impede alcohol policies' success.

For each of the case studies, relevant historical background is given first before an overview of the policy itself. A section on theories and contexts follows, assessing whether the ideas presented in Chapters 3 and 4 offer insight into the case study. Finally the key lessons of the case study are explored, illustrating what contemporary researchers and policymakers can learn from an often-overlooked—but deeply prescient—historical example of an effort to change alcohol policy.

---

1 For a discussion of different interpretations of American Prohibition's successes and failures see Zimring and Hawkins (1992, pp. 67–9).

Soviet Union in the 1980s

Historical Background

In order to understand the historical context of the first case study—an effort to sharply decrease alcohol consumption in the Soviet Union in the 1980s—it is necessary to briefly explore the history of alcohol consumption in Russia. This history is long and complex, and is the subject of a growing body of valuable research. As Smith and Christian (1984, p. 309) have reported, in the early twentieth century overall per capita alcohol consumption in Russia was quite moderate relative to many other European countries. Specifically, statistics suggest that per capita consumption in Russia was only slightly higher than in Sweden and was less than a quarter of per capita consumption in France. However, as Smith and Christian have outlined, rather than consuming this alcohol in regular moderation, in much of the countryside from the nineteenth century through the early twentieth century "peasants confined their drinking to a few festive occasions on which they drank to oblivion" (p. 309).

During the First World War, to ensure that alcohol use did not disrupt the war effort, Tsar Nicholas II effectively introduced prohibition in Russia, as only a small selection of establishments were allowed to sell alcohol; this policy remained in force long after the tsarist regime had fallen (Krasnov, 2003, p. 15). Interestingly, the policy was adopted despite the lack of an influential temperance movement in Russia at that time (Schrad, 2010, pp. 7–9). Prohibition was affirmed in the aftermath of the Bolshevik Revolution in order to preserve dwindling grain supplies (as described in Transchel, 2006, p. 70). However, in 1930, seeing an opportunity to increase governmental revenue, Stalin mandated that vodka production be increased and brought under the government's purview (Herlihy, 2002; Osokina, 2001, p. 219, note 11). Stalin made this change even though he was personally affected by alcohol's social harms—his father was an alcoholic and one of his sons died from causes related to alcoholism (McNeal, 1990, p. 162). With the energy of the state behind production efforts, between 1940 and 1985 the sale of alcohol in the Soviet Union increased more than seven-fold (as cited in Herlihy, 2002, p. 154). More specifically, during the 1970s, Soviet production of spirits, including vodka, increased by a third even though the population only grew by nine percent (Klose, 1979). Alongside these increases in consumption, alcohol-related public harms ostensibly rose as well. Although statements from 1950s Soviet reports that "70 percent of all crimes" were committed by intoxicated individuals cannot be taken at face value, they indicate the perceived pervasiveness of alcohol-related crime (as quoted in Connor, 1979, p. 439). Yet efforts targeting certain aspects of problematic drinking—such as penalties for public drunkenness that were instituted in the 1960s—seemed to do little to reduce alcohol's harmful impacts (Transchel, 2003).

Case Study

By the 1980s, alcohol's social harms exerted a large toll on the USSR. Alcohol consumption was responsible for a 10–20 percent reduction in industrial productivity (Farrell, 1990), and it was now suggested that more than 75 percent of murders were said to be committed by intoxicated offenders (Anderson and Hibbs, 1992, p. 442). Alcohol's negative impacts were exacerbated by the lack of services available to alcoholics in search of recovery. A 1981 report by US-based academics, for example, noted that although the Soviet public was generally sympathetic toward individuals with alcohol problems, "scholars and officials alike—especially those in the medical community … generally express impatience, irritation, anger, or outright contempt for men and women who abuse alcohol" (Field and Powell, 1981, p. 41).

In the late spring of 1985, just two months after becoming general secretary of the Communist Party, Mikhail Gorbachev began a landmark campaign to significantly reduce alcohol consumption in the Soviet Union (Herlihy, 2002, p. 154). Gorbachev's campaign utilized a variety of different tactics, including urging people to consume non-alcoholic drinks, increasing vodka prices, and shutting vodka distilleries (Vågerö, 2011, p. 20). A minimum drinking age of 21 was implemented and alcohol advertising was forbidden (Baltagi and Geishecker, 2006, p. 893). The campaign's efforts to control alcohol were so extreme that one commentator has labeled the campaign "semi-prohibition" (Vågerö, 2011, p. 20), meriting the inclusion of this dramatic policy shift within this chapter.

In the short term, by some measures, the campaign was successful, as state production of vodka and wine fell by more than half between 1980 and 1988 (Transchel, 2003, p. 582). Sales of alcohol also declined by more than 60 percent between 1984 and 1987, according to another estimate (Farrell, 1990). In addition to these declines in consumption, some alcohol-related social harms also fell. Between 1984 and 1988, for example, suicides declined by more than a third and violent deaths declined by more than a quarter—decreases that observers have linked to the reductions in alcohol consumption (Cook, 2007, p. 92).

These short-term declines, however, were not sustained. By 1991 alcohol consumption had almost risen to pre-1985 levels once again (Nemtsov, 2011, p. 41). Additionally, the campaign produced new social harms of its own. The scarcity of alcohol meant that queues outside alcohol outlets were often quite long—sometimes comprising thousands of people—and the frustration in these queues sometimes produced violence (Kondakov, 1988). On New Year's Day, 1991, for instance, the scarcity of alcohol prompted a particularly destructive riot in Siberia (Herlihy, 2002, p. 156).

Another social harm associated with the campaign was a rise in deaths and injuries due to the consumption of homebrewed alcohol (or moonshine). According to one estimate, in 1988 some 11,000 people in the Soviet Union died as a result of drinking industrial alcohol and other homemade alcoholic beverages; some of these beverages were made from perfume and toothpaste, which contained alcohol at the time ("Prohibition, Soviet style", 1990). Of course, consumption of moonshine had also occurred in earlier eras; data sets from the 1920s and the 1950s, for example, indicate that illegal distilling was also widespread (Connor, 1979, p. 435). However, Gorbachev's campaign against alcohol did lead to increased demand for homemade brews, and so many people resorted to making their own alcohol during this period that sugar supplies actually dwindled, negatively affecting non-drinkers as well (Associated Press, 1990).

Although the campaign initially enjoyed some public support—particularly from women (Partanen, 1993, p. 130S)—it became increasingly unpopular. Indeed, as Nemtsov (2011, p. 41) has explained, it produced "a unanimity never before seen in Soviet popular resistance" as people banded together to create their own alcohol and undermine the government's effort. The government's effort conflicted with several prominent cultural attitudes. In particular, alcohol consumption was traditionally seen in some quarters as part of a masculine male identity (Herlihy, 2002; Hinote, Cockerham, and Abbott, 2009, p. 1255)—a difficult cultural roadblock for the anti-alcohol campaigners to overcome. Ultimately, the campaign's massive unpopularity and the loss of government revenues from alcohol sales it engendered meant that, by 1988, its influence began to wane and some of its restrictions were relaxed (Treml, 1997, p. 229).

Theories and Contexts

When exploring the question of whether the theories presented in Chapters 3 and 4 offer insight into this case study, it is important to note that Chapter 3's policymaking frameworks were primarily developed to explain policymaking in democracies. Issues of public support, consideration of research evidence, and the importance of elections often do not exert the same influence in undemocratic contexts. Gorbachev's decision to press ahead with the campaign was certainly undemocratic; as described above, the campaign proved increasingly unpopular with the public and also lacked support from some key governmental officials. In particular, the Ministry of Trade and the Ministry of Finance were both initially opposed to the campaign since it would reduce their revenues (Herlihy, 2002, p. 154). It is intriguing to note that Gorbachev's campaign was not the first example of such undemocratic alcohol policymaking in Russia. As Schrad (2010, p. 144) has observed, Gorbachev's actions mirrored those of Tsar Nicholas II, who pursued the unpopular prohibition effort during World War I that was discussed earlier in this chapter. Although the Tsar's decision had a different explicit motivation, as it was undertaken to ensure that alcohol use did not disrupt the war effort (Krasnov, 2003), both historical examples featured leaders pressing ahead with dramatic changes in alcohol policy.

The example of Gorbachev's autocratic campaign illustrates the importance of recognizing that alcohol policies are made within a very wide range of different political contexts. The fact that many of Chapter 3's theories were developed in a democratic context highlights the need for more theories of alcohol policymaking in non-democratic settings in order to achieve a truly global understanding of the forces that shape alcohol policy.

Despite this different context, though, several ideas presented in Chapter 4 seem to offer insight into the emergence—and ostensible failure—of Gorbachev's anti-alcohol campaign. In particular, Chapter 4's emphasis on the importance of historical and political contexts in shaping reactions to alcohol policy is borne out in this case study. Specifically, Schrad (2010, pp. 144–5) has observed that public opinion about the campaign became increasingly negative just as *glasnost* was beginning to gain ground; the loosening of some restrictions during these years meant that people were able to express themselves more freely—and thus were better able to articulate their dissatisfaction with the government's anti-alcohol campaign. This idea that political and historical contexts—in particular, *glasnost*—shaped reactions to alcohol policies thus supports Chapter 4's emphasis on these contexts' importance.

A second theme outlined in Chapter 4 was the centrality of public opinion to policy discussions regarding alcohol. In studies of public opinion data from two different countries, Giesbrecht and colleagues (2007) and Greenfield and colleagues (2007) found that policies that limited the availability of alcohol were generally less popular with the public than other types of alcohol policies. Thus it is not surprising that in the Soviet Union a campaign to severely limit the availability of alcohol lacked public support.

On a related theme, Chapter 4 also demonstrated that public opinion can often be instrumental in facilitating the adoption and implementation of alcohol policies. Johnson and colleagues' (2004) work, cited in that chapter, discussed how a lack of public support helped explain why proposals to increase national excise taxes on alcohol in the US in the 1990s, were not adopted. Although Gorbachev's anti-alcohol policies *were* adopted by the USSR's autocratic government, the lack of public support for these policies—shown by individuals' efforts to create their own illicit alcoholic beverages—likely illustrates why they did not succeed in achieving their long-term goals.

Finally, researchers have found that influential organized groups can foment and mobilize public support for alcohol policies, as explored in detail in the previous chapter. This same theme can also be identified in the Soviet Union example, as Gorbachev clearly recognized the importance of such organized groups. Indeed, Herlihy (2002) has detailed how, as one of the first components of his campaign, Gorbachev created an organized group to support the policy: the All-Union Voluntary Temperance Promotion Society. (This society was only "voluntary" in an Orwellian sense since its initial core membership consisted of bureaucrats and loyal members of the Communist Party.) According to Herlihy, one of the organization's main goals was to inspire the development of local "civic organisations" that would move the campaign forward, and through these local groups, the society was eventually able to claim some 14 million members (pp. 154–5). Gorbachev's attempt to use organized groups to facilitate the adoption and implementation of anti-alcohol policies shows a clear recognition of the potential power of such groups in alcohol policymaking.

Key Lessons

The lessons and implications of Gorbachev's anti-alcohol campaign—and its ostensible failures—are numerous. First and foremost, its similarities with Tsar Nicholas II's effort more than 70 years earlier (Schrad, 2010) show how concerns about excessive consumption, and the tactics that governments employ to reduce that consumption, can be remarkably similar over time. (The potential for excessive consumption to hinder the war effort helped motivate the Tsar's decision [Krasnov, 2003]). Even in more recent times, excessive alcohol consumption remains a concern in Russia. In 1995, for example, a decade after Gorbachev began his anti-alcohol campaign, Boris Yeltsin responded to significant increases in the amount of European vodka that was being imported into Russia by introducing restrictive quotas on such imports—a measure that once again encouraged the underground production of alcoholic beverages (Herlihy, 2002, p. 159). Similarly, an effort in 2000 in Russia to raise alcohol taxes by 40 percent "provoked long lines outside distilleries and prompted regional governments to refuse to implement the new taxes, fearing civil disobedience" (Baltagi and Geishecker, 2006, p. 893). Nevertheless, despite these similarities, concerns and campaigns are not *identical* across time; instead, they are also shaped by the specific political and historical contexts in which they emerge. In particular, this case study shows how a very dramatic political and historical moment—the *glasnost* era—influenced reactions to Gorbachev's campaign (Schrad, 2010).

The second key lesson taught by this case study is that many themes related to alcohol policymaking have cross-cultural resonance. In the West, the failings of early-twentieth-century American Prohibition are well known, and much has been written about the many high-powered criminals and ordinary people alike who sought to evade the law through illegal imports or moonshine (Aaron and Musto, 1981; Zimring and Hawkins, 1992). The Soviet Union's drive to sharply reduce alcohol use is less well known in the West than American Prohibition, but the two policies produced very similar results. Alcohol-related social harms may have declined during the early years of Gorbachev's campaign (Cook, 2007), but as with American Prohibition the unpopularity of the campaign—and the mass production of moonshine it encouraged—helped lead to its abandonment.

Further similarities can also be identified in the *aftermath* of these two historical examples. Specifically, in the years following American Prohibition and Gorbachev's campaign, the same pattern of alcohol consumption can be seen. As already described, in the initial period after Gorbachev's campaign was instituted, sales of alcohol fell dramatically (Farrell, 1990), yet by 1991 alcohol consumption had nearly returned to pre-1985 levels (Nemtsov, 2011, p. 41). Similarly, following Prohibition's implementation in the US, alcohol consumption initially declined dramatically, but in later years began to rise again (Miron and Zwiebel, 1991).

Although these two policy movements were unique, their similar results suggest that some knowledge about alcohol and alcohol policy has cross-cultural and cross-national applicability.

The third and final key lesson to discuss here is the importance of considering the wide variety of political contexts in which alcohol policies are made. Many of the policy frameworks described in Chapter 3 were developed in a democratic context, yet Gorbachev's decision, like many other decisions about alcohol policy, emerged in an undemocratic setting. Although some themes discussed in Chapter 4—such as the importance of political and historical contexts—also seem to apply to this case study of undemocratic policymaking, more specific research and theoretical work on alcohol policymaking in non-democratic arenas is needed.

Sri Lanka in the Early Twentieth Century

Historical Background

This chapter's second case study focuses on efforts to adopt prohibition-like policies in Sri Lanka in the early twentieth century. The majority of Sri Lankans are adherents of Buddhism—a religion in which the consumption of intoxicating substances is seen as an impediment to enlightenment (Oldstone-Moore, 2003, p. 120). Therefore it is perhaps not surprising that literature from the era prior to European colonization of the island contained few mentions of alcohol usage; indeed, it is clear that alcohol did not play a central role in pre-colonial culture (Samarasinghe, 2006).

In the nineteenth century, however, the British colonial administration harmonized a government monopoly system to control alcohol retail; this monopoly system persisted into the early twentieth century—the time period considered in this case study—and became economically powerful (Rogers, 1989, pp. 321–2). Seizing upon these facts, in the twentieth century many temperance advocates and other commentators in Sri Lanka argued that consuming alcohol was a harmful *foreign* practice, associated with European colonialists and Christianity (Berkwitz, 2006; Rogers, 1989, p. 324). This emphasis on the "foreignness" of alcohol echoes concerns about the "foreignness" of gin that were voiced during the eighteenth-century British gin craze, described at the beginning of Chapter 4.

Case Study

The focus of this case study is two powerful temperance campaigns spearheaded by native Sri Lankans in 1904 and 1912. Neither movement was successful in achieving its goal of instituting national prohibition, but each impacted Sri Lankan society greatly and left an important legacy for future debates about alcohol policy.

The 1904 campaign was led by educated Sri Lankan elites who were able to make their voices heard and gain influence by championing the cause of temperance. Specifically, according to Rogers (1989, p. 332), for these local elites the 1904 movement "served as a means to formulate indirectly a social and cultural identity apart from that provided by the colonial state. In this guise it enabled politically powerless groups to seize positions of social leadership." In other words, for some Sri Lankans, the campaign had positive and important political and social consequences, although, as already described, it did not achieve its ultimate goal. Despite its legacy of empowering some Sri Lankan elites, the 1904 movement never represented a significant opposition to the national, colonial status quo. Nevertheless this "failure" allowed the 1912 temperance campaign to come into being; this campaign focused on the same concerns and used many of the same tactics, but represented a more significant challenge.

The 1912 temperance campaign quickly became aligned to a wider political movement against British colonialism. As Bond (1988, p. 62) has detailed, campaigners framed alcohol as a corrupting Western import, and abstinence—which deprived the colonial authorities of revenues from government-monopolized alcohol sales—was promoted as an act of anti-imperial resistance. Like the 1904 campaign, this later movement also offered many educated Sri Lankans opportunities to express themselves and gain influence (de Silva, 1981). Colonial authorities recognized that the temperance campaign constituted a real threat—much more so than the earlier campaign (Kannangara, 1984). As de Silva (1981, pp. 376–7) has explained, initially the authorities tried to ban village leaders from joining temperance organizations; however, the public outcry against this move was so great, both in Sri Lanka and in Britain, that the policy was abandoned. This abandonment was treated as a victory by temperance leaders and further strengthened the movement's power. However, in 1915 riots broke out and the British declared martial law (De Mel, 2001, p. 14). The government blamed these riots on the temperance campaigners—even though most rioters *were not* actually drawn from the movement itself (Kannangara, 1984). Nevertheless, the movement's power base was fatally eroded when many prominent Buddhists were arrested and some temperance workers were even killed in the aftermath of the riots (Peebles, 2006, p. 81).

Theories and Contexts

Several of the ideas presented in chapters 3 and 4 offer insights into the key themes raised in this case study. The first theme that merits discussion here is the deeply political aspect of both movements—and of the 1912 movement in particular. As discussed above, both movements framed alcohol and its social harms as examples of colonialism's ills, thus linking temperance with political resistance to colonial rule (Bond, 1988; Rogers, 1989). More dramatically, the 1912 movement forged deep links with a wider political wave of resistance to colonialism—a threat that was taken seriously by the British (de Silva, 1981). This emphasis on forging links with growing political movements reflects Kingdon's (2003) idea—discussed in Chapter 3—that a sympathetic *political* climate is necessary for an issue to arise onto the agenda. In Sri Lanka, the ability of campaigners to seize upon the anti-colonial political climate pervasive at the time likely facilitated their success in making temperance a prominent topic in national debates.

Additionally, the tendency of campaigners to frame alcohol as foreign and symbolic of colonialism shows how alcohol policy and attitudes to alcohol can be shaped by historical and political factors—a theme also evidenced in other countries' historical experiences with alcohol. Chapter 4 cited the example of South Africa, where drinking and congregating in shebeens (or illegal alcohol outlets) became associated with resistance to apartheid from the 1950s onward (Parry, 2005). Although these two examples are inverses of each other—in Sri Lanka temperance was associated with political resistance, whilst in South Africa it was consumption—they both highlight how attitudes to alcohol can be linked with wider concerns.

One final point to consider about the political aspects of the 1904 and 1912 movements is the influence they gave to some Sri Lankan elites. Acting as the "policy entrepreneurs" described in Kingdon's (2003, pp. 180–82) theory, such elites seized upon problems present in Sri Lankan society—namely, alcohol's social harms—and presented temperance-focused policy solutions. These social elites often had few other opportunities to exert true influence and political leadership under colonial rule. Interestingly, as Rogers (1989) has noted, temperance movements in other parts of the world were also led by similar societal groups—namely, individuals who maintained some privileges in their societies, but were formally excluded from full participation in political or economic life. Other examples cited by Rogers include women in the US and middle-class blacks in South Africa who also played key roles in organized temperance efforts.

A second theme that stands out from this case study is the role of religion. The early twentieth century temperance movement in Sri Lanka had naturally strong links with Buddhist traditions since, as discussed earlier, the consumption of intoxicating substances is seen as an impediment to enlightenment in Buddhism, and therefore often frowned upon (Oldstone-Moore, 2003). Buddhism played such a strong, animating role in the 1904 campaign that Sri Lanka's Catholic minority was reluctant to join the movement (Rogers, 1989). Buddhist groups and Buddhist precepts similarly were central to the 1912 campaign (Bond, 1988), and in 1956 a Buddhist revivalist movement in Sri Lanka helped spur calls for the national adoption of prohibition; this effort was also unsuccessful, however (Harvey, 2000).

One can identify a religious element in other temperance movements in other parts of the world. For example, the temperance movements that emerged in Europe and the US during the early twentieth century were often rooted in Protestant values (McTighe, 1994; Phelan, 2011; Tyrrell, 1991), while Islamic precepts against alcohol consumption continue to influence low rates of alcohol consumption in Muslim-majority countries (WHO, 2004a). Similarly, Chapter 4 raised the example of the US state of Utah—home to the headquarters of the Mormon Church—which has traditionally maintained more restrictive alcohol policies than many other US states. Such examples illustrate religion's potential to help shape not only temperance movements, but also attitudes toward alcohol and alcohol policies more generally.

A third and final theme related to the case study is the use of evidence in the temperance campaigns. In 1904, campaigners deployed medical evidence at rallies to highlight the detrimental long-term health effects of alcohol consumption; they also worked hard to emphasize alcohol's links with crime (Rogers, 1989). Although the rigor and accuracy of some of the evidence deployed by campaigners might not withstand contemporary scrutiny, the use of evidence *at all* to drive policy-related campaigns is an important development. By focusing on such medical evidence, some Sri Lankan campaigners went further than the campaigners during the eighteenth-century British "gin craze," who had also tried to link excessive gin consumption to poor health, crime, infant mortality, and other social harms (Dillon, 2002; Porter, 1985). Although it would be a stretch to interpret the Sri Lankan campaigners' efforts as proto-public health campaigns, it is important to note their emphasis on calculating and describing alcohol's social harms, which emerged several decades before a significant research base about these harms developed in the mid-to-late twentieth century.

Key Lessons

One of the most fundamental lessons that can be gleaned from this case study is that historical alcohol-related movements can leave a long legacy. Indeed, the temperance campaigns that were launched more than a hundred years ago are sometimes still cited in contemporary debates about alcohol policy in Sri Lanka ("Temperance and compassion", 2010). A number of "programmes and press conferences" about drugs' harms were scheduled for July 2012 to mark the 100th anniversary of the Sri Lanka Temperance Association's founding and its 1912 campaign ("Media can make great change ...", 2011). Just as Buddhism played a central role in the 1904 and 1912 campaigns, contemporary efforts to educate the public about alcohol's social harms are often led by Buddhist monks; some of these recent campaigns have even employed rhetoric similar to that used in the earlier efforts, with one monk campaigner telling a reporter in 2008: "The British colonial rulers promoted alcohol to destroy the local culture and traditional values" (as quoted in Seneviratne, 2008). This perspective—that alcohol was foreign and a tool of colonial rule—was, as discussed above, a centerpiece of the 1912 temperance movement. Interestingly, however, the popular attitude toward following the Buddhist precepts against alcohol consumption may have changed in more recent times. As Oldstone-Moore (2003, p. 121) has argued, today in Sri Lanka "strict adherence to the Buddhist precepts is seen as a mark of the unworldly and non-elite; drinking alcohol is a mark of higher social status." This development shows that consumption is itself subject to historical contexts and affected by changes over time.

From the 1980s through the 2000s a civil war between the Sri Lankan government and the Liberation Tigers of Tamil Eelam drew much governmental attention and resources. In 2000, Médecins Sans Frontières conducted a survey of people displaced by the violence, finding that 11 percent had been victims of torture and more than a third had experienced the death of a close friend or relative in the conflict (de Jong et al., 2002). The magnitude of these war-related harms further burdened the already-overstretched resources of the hospitals and local authorities in the conflict's hot spots, likely restricting the amount of resources available for alcohol's social harms. Yet, as campaigners pointed out in the 2000s, almost as many Sri Lankans died each year as a result of alcohol- and tobacco-related causes as had died in the entire civil war (Seneviratne, 2008).

More recently, as the violence has subsided, efforts have once again been taken to reduce alcohol's social harms. In 2006, new legislation was adopted which forbade the retail of alcohol through self-service vending machines and also established a minimum legal drinking age of 21 ("New legislation in Sri Lanka", 2006). The act took years to pass and its legality was challenged in the Supreme Court; however its eventual adoption and implementation was aided by non-governmental organizations (NGOs), scientific groups, and youth groups who drew upon research evidence about alcohol's harms and prevention efforts other countries had adopted. One youth group even secured 50,000 signatures in favor of the bill ("New legislation in Sri Lanka", 2006). The fact that research evidence seems to have played a role in the passage of the act offers support for Weiss' (1982) idea, outlined in Chapter 3, that research evidence *can* impact policy under certain conditions; the role of the youth movement and organized groups in encouraging adoption of the law also mirrors Weiss' (1983) insights about the importance of competing interests in the policy process. Encouragingly, in 2007, the year after the act's passage, liquor consumption in Sri Lanka fell by more than 9 percent, according to the country's deputy finance minister (although some critics disagreed and alleged consumption had actually increased) ("Liquor consumption falls ...", 2009).

A second key lesson to take away from this case study is a further reminder that movements to change alcohol policy can reflect larger political concerns. Many of Sri Lanka's early temperance campaigners did not merely focus on limiting access to alcohol—they focused on framing alcohol as a symbol of colonialism and abstinence as a means of resistance to British rule. These movements therefore often contained an essential *political* dimension. Thus, when analyzing efforts to change alcohol policy, it is essential to examine whether these efforts are connected to broader social and political movements. A similar theme can also be detected in the Soviet Union example, where one should consider the role of *glasnost*—and the political and social climate it fostered—in boosting public resistance to the anti-alcohol campaign (Schrad, 2010, pp. 144–5).

A third and final lesson to consider is that, like alcohol policies themselves, alcohol-related social movements can rarely be transported wholesale across countries. Instead, such movements need to adapt to local cultural and political contexts. This lesson can be seen in the fact that although Protestant missionaries endeavored to encourage temperance in Sri Lanka in the late nineteenth century, these early temperance movements failed to gain prominence; indeed, temperance ideas did not achieve real influence until they were promoted within a Buddhist framework by native Sri Lankans (Rogers, 1989). Sri Lanka's experience is similar to that of Sweden, where an attempt during the early nineteenth century to create a temperance organization closely resembling an American model was not successful (Bengtsson, 1938, p. 134). Indeed, as described in Chapter 4, Schrad (2010) has persuasively argued that although emergent temperance movements in the early twentieth century were influenced by similar campaigns in other countries, many such campaigns were adapted to fit local contexts and societies' unique political structures.

More recently, similar concerns about the need to adapt alcohol policies to fit local contexts and political structures have been directly raised in Sri Lanka. In 2006, a medical expert at the University of Colombo wrote in the journal *Addiction* that, on the issue of alcohol's social harms, "successful responses implemented by other countries, for example in Europe, sometimes *but not always* offer ready-made routes for Sri Lanka to follow" (Samarasinghe, 2006, p. 628) (emphasis added). This stress on the importance of adapting policies to suit local contexts matches Dolowitz and Marsh's (2000) landmark findings about impediments to policy diffusion that were discussed in Chapter 3.

Related to this issue is the more specific concern that alcohol policies must reflect developing countries' unique circumstances and characteristics. The same Sri Lankan medical expert cited in the previous paragraph identified the need for alcohol policies to address the harms caused by both legally- and illegally-produced alcohol, since much of the alcohol consumed in some developing countries falls into the latter category (Samarasinghe, 2006, p. 626). Indeed, the important role that illicit alcohol can play in segments of Sri Lankan society has even been the subject of a recent monograph (Gamburd, 2008). An additional concern that other commentary has identified is the role of the alcohol industry in promoting alcohol consumption in developing countries such as Sri Lanka ("New legislation in Sri Lanka", 2006). This theme connects directly to the discussion in Chapter 4 about the differences between alcohol policymaking in developed and developing countries. In particular, Bakke and Endal's (2010) research—cited in Chapter 4's discussion—shows that concerns about the multinational alcohol industry's attempts to influence policy in developing countries are not wholly unfounded.

Conclusion

Although much research has examined the adoption and implications of Prohibition in the early-twentieth-century US, this chapter has shown that other less-studied efforts to sharply reduce alcohol consumption also offer valuable lessons. Such lessons include the importance of political factors in shaping movements to change alcohol policy and the long historical legacies that such movements can have. Indeed, it is important to recognize that temperance movements and policy efforts to dramatically curtail consumption have gained influence in numerous countries around the world. In the late nineteenth and early twentieth centuries alone, as detailed in Chapter 3, temperance movements flourished not only in the US and Sri Lanka but also in the UK, Australia, and Canada (Blainey, 2003; Morone, 2003; "The hemisphere", 1959).

How similar were these various efforts and campaigns? Like American Prohibition, Gorbachev's campaign and the early-twentieth-century movements in Sri Lanka can both be seen as "failures." Gorbachev's campaign did not produce long-lasting decreases in alcohol consumption, while the Sri Lankan movements did not achieve national adoption of prohibition. Religion played an important role in both the American and the Sri Lankan movements—although the specific religions involved differed. Negative public reactions also stymied both the American and Soviet policies (Aaron and Musto, 1981).

Even the Sri Lankan and Soviet case studies themselves share some similarities. One such similarity is the role of stereotypes in impeding efforts to reduce alcohol consumption. Specifically, in both Sri Lanka and Russia, a stereotype exists in some areas which asserts that, for men, alcohol consumption is an essential component of masculinity. One can see evidence of this stereotype in the fact that in Sri Lanka today, men consume the overwhelming majority of alcohol, and, as Gamburd (2008) has shown, consumption is often seen as a social activity central to masculine identity. Similarly, in Soviet society, one factor that was said to hinder efforts to reduce alcohol consumption was the belief among many men that consumption proved their masculinity (Herlihy, 2002; Hinote, Cockerham, and Abbott, 2009). Specific concern about young men's drinking levels remains high even today in Sri Lanka, as "alcohol use disproportionately harms Sri Lankan males" (Perera and Torabi, 2009, p. 2408).

One final question to consider is *why* these movements and policies "failed." Many potential explanations have already been outlined, including the lack of public support for Gorbachev's campaign in the Soviet Union and the opposition of the British colonial authorities in Sri Lanka to the 1912 movement. As noted above, after Sri Lanka gained independence in the mid twentieth century and overcame the 1983–2009 civil war, the country *did* adopt a policy strategy to combat alcohol's social harms. The alcohol policies that were adopted did not include total prohibition, but many matched the evidence-based policy recommendations the WHO subsequently put forward in its Global Strategy, which was discussed in Chapter 1 ("New legislation in Sri Lanka", 2006).

In addition to the explanations already discussed, another reason for the Soviet "failure" could be the infeasibility of prohibition (or a prohibition-esque policy) itself. Some critics—such as the commentator cited in Chapter 1 who, in response to the Pine Ridge case argued that Prohibition "didn't work in the United States in the 1920s and it is not working for the Sioux people today" (Newman, 2012)—

would likely agree with this argument. The Soviet Union example illustrates that prohibition-esque policies can be undermined by the illegal production of alcohol. Whether Sri Lanka would have faced such problems is impossible to know, but the current presence of illegally-produced alcohol in Sri Lanka certainly brings this question to the forefront (Gamburd, 2008; Samarasinghe, 2006).

A related but more nuanced explanation for the "failure" of the Soviet campaign and other efforts for dramatic policy change can perhaps be found in Lindblom's (1959; 1979) theory of incrementalism, which posits that policymaking is typically an incremental process consisting of small steps rather than revolutionary changes. Lindblom's theory does indeed offer insight into alcohol policymaking; as discussed in Chapter 4, Thamarangsi (2008) has argued that incrementalism explains some aspects of alcohol policymaking in Thailand in the 1990s and 2000s. Perhaps Lindblom's theory can offer insight not only into policy adoption but also into policy *implementation*. Like policymakers, members of the public who must adhere to alcohol policies and governmental bureaucrats who must enforce those policies might also be less willing to accept dramatic policy changes such as prohibition. This inability could explain the difficulties governments face when trying to sustain public support for these policies, and when endeavoring to ensure they are enforced. Ultimately, the question of whether prohibition and other dramatic policy changes are inherently unworkable—an issue that is at the heart of this chapter—is deeply divisive, but essential to debate in any investigation of alcohol policymaking.

Chapter 6
General Efforts to Reduce
Alcohol's Social Harms

Prohibition is of course not the only approach societies have taken to reduce alcohol's overall social harms. Less restrictive policies have also been introduced in an attempt to target consumption and thus decrease alcohol's burden on society. Do similar factors explain both the adoption of prohibition-type strategies and of more general policies? What role does evidence play in debates about these kinds of policies? This chapter aims to answer these and other questions by exploring two further case studies: Sweden's state-run alcohol retail monopoly, and the UK's cultural traditions of consumption in rounds and pints. As in the last chapter, these case studies are used to evaluate the utility of the ideas advanced in chapters 3 and 4, as well as to illuminate lessons about alcohol policymaking.

All of the policy changes and debates discussed in this chapter took place in more recent times than the campaigns discussed in the previous chapter. Thus, unlike Gorbachev's anti-alcohol effort in the Soviet Union and the early twentieth century temperance movements in Sri Lanka, the case studies in this chapter belong to a time when the *public health* approach to alcohol was dominant. As outlined in Chapter 2, this approach aims to prevent or mitigate health issues that arise from alcohol consumption in the *overall population* and endeavors not to stigmatize individual drinkers; the approach has gained prominence since the 1970s and is now among the most important frameworks for understanding, and combating, alcohol misuse (Bruun et al., 1975; Tigerstedt, 1999). Within the public health approach a significant "what works" literature has developed about the best ways to prevent and reduce alcohol's social harms (e.g., Babor et al., 2010). The existence of this vast literature—previously explored in more detail in Chapter 2—means that the policies and proposals discussed here emerged at a time when research evidence was gaining greater societal attention.

Alcohol Policy in Sweden

This chapter's first case study illustrates how many of the larger forces outlined in Chapter 4—such as globalization and political changes—can impact alcohol policies. The case study focuses on Sweden's experiences in the 1990s and the early 2000s, when its traditionally restrictive alcohol policies were challenged by increasing European integration.

In order to understand the significance of this challenge it is necessary to first explore Sweden's history of restrictive alcohol policies and powerful temperance movements. Indeed, in the 1800s and early 1900s, temperance movements exerted considerable influence in Sweden and at their height around 1910 more than 375,000 Swedes belonged to such organizations (Bengtsson, 1938, p. 136; "Temperance in Sweden", 1853). Given that Sweden's population reached 5.5 million in that year (Ljungmark, 1979, p. 29), this means that nearly 7 percent of the population were members of temperance groups. By the early twentieth century, many of these organizations called for the implementation of outright prohibition—a policy that was not only implemented in the US during this period, but also in Sweden's neighbors Norway and Finland (Schrad, 2010). Additionally, as discussed in the previous chapter, prohibition was also adopted in the nearby country of Russia during World War I (Transchel, 2006).

Prohibition became such a salient issue in Sweden that in 1909 temperance leaders arranged an unofficial referendum on the subject, and just over 55 percent of all Swedish adults signed a petition in favor of outlawing "all alcoholic beverages, stronger than light beer" (Nycander, 1998, p. 17). The government did not immediately act upon this popular endorsement, however, instead choosing to follow a compromise proposal advanced by Ivan Bratt, a doctor in Stockholm (Shanks and Tilley, 1987, pp. 193–4). In many ways, Bratt prefigured more recent public health alcohol experts as he believed that alcohol policymaking should be informed by rigorous scientific and medical evidence (Eriksen, 2003). Bratt's position as a doctor allowed him to focus public attention on the health aspects of the alcohol debate (Alexius, Castillo, and Rosenström, 2011, p. 13). Although Bratt did not advocate outright prohibition, he recognized alcohol's great potential as a driver of social harms, writing: "The fight against human excesses … is difficult. The fight against profiteering purveyors of alcohol is difficult. The fight against these two Powers combined is HOPELESS" (as quoted in "Sweden: Bratt Resigns", 1928).

Bratt proposed that, instead of prohibition, adult Swedes could be given ration books limiting their ability to procure alcoholic spirits—a policy that would presumably ensure that alcohol was kept out of the hands of individuals with a history of criminal behavior or alcohol problems, since the ration allocated to each individual "depended on various factors such as gender, social and marital status and social stability" (Mäkelä, Rossow, and Tryggvesson, 2002, p. 14).[1] In 1919, this ration-book system that Bratt proposed was enshrined into law (Shanks and Tilley, 1987, p. 194). Several years later, in 1922, an official referendum on prohibition in Sweden only found 49 percent of voters were now in favor—a percentage lower than that found in the unofficial 1909 petition, and an amount much less than the two-thirds majority required to adopt prohibition (Schrad, 2010,

---

1 Shanks and Tilley (1987, p. 195) have argued that these criteria were "grossly discriminatory," as women, residents of rural areas, and people with lower incomes typically received smaller rations.

p. 102). The ration-book system that Bratt pioneered remained in place for more than three decades. In 1955, however, faced with declining public support, the system was eventually discontinued, and public drunkenness in Sweden doubled over the next two years (Nycander, 1998, p. 24; "Rigid temperance laws ...", 1967).

Although the ration-book system has long since disappeared, Sweden maintains another alcohol policy that has roots in the nineteenth century: that of a state-controlled alcohol monopoly (Bilefsky, 2007). Sweden's monopoly consists of two parts: a state-owned production monopoly known as Vin och Sprit and a state-controlled retail monopoly known as the Systembolaget (Kurzer, 2001; Shanks and Tilley, 1987, p. 194). The Systembolaget is today one of the world's best-known and most comprehensive alcohol retail monopolies. As well as facilitating greater government control over the public's access to alcohol and higher revenue for the government from alcohol sales, the goal of the Systembolaget is also to remove the profit motive from alcohol retail, giving retailers less incentive to encourage greater consumption (Doos, 1982). Although some low-strength beverages—3.5 percent ABV or less—can be sold in food stores, stronger beverages can only be sold in Systembolaget-controlled shops ("Privatizing Sweden's retail ...", 2010; "Rigid temperance laws ...", 1967). These shops are typically plainly-decorated and unassuming (de Castella, 2012) and have traditionally maintained more restricted opening hours and steeper prices than alcohol shops in other European countries (Bevanger, 2005).

In addition to the persistence of this monopoly, the mid twentieth century also witnessed the introduction of a range of additional measures designed to reduce alcohol's social harms in Sweden. For example, by 1960 high taxes had been instituted on alcohol to reduce overall consumption (Nycander, 1998), and during the 1970s random breath tests were implemented to reduce alcohol-impaired driving among Swedes (Davies and Walsh, 1983, p. 201). In 1979, wine and liquor advertisements were prohibited altogether (Doos, 1982). Perhaps not surprisingly, given this range of restrictions, during the 1970s Swedish alcohol consumption rates actually fell—in sharp contrast to trends in many other European countries during that time period (Davies and Walsh, 1983, p. 213). During the 1980s, death rates from liver cirrhosis in Sweden also generally declined (Selvanathan and Selvanathan, 2005, pp. 289–90). (Researchers have linked the more long-term fall in deaths due to liver disease from the 1970s through the 1990s to declining spirits sales [Stokkeland et al., 2006]). In the early 1980s the Systembolaget spearheaded a campaign to discourage drinking, employing members of the pop group Abba, while at the same time high taxes remained in place on alcoholic beverages (Doos, 1982). By the mid 1990s, alcohol taxes constituted 6 percent of the total tax bill in Sweden—a figure even more impressive when one considers Sweden's reputation as an overall high-tax country (McIvor and Tucker, 1997). Indeed, during this period, a bottle of spirits was typically more than twice as expensive in Sweden relative to France (Daley, 2001).

Kurzer (2001) has explored why Sweden has traditionally maintained such restrictive alcohol policies, observing that Sweden's social democratic philosophy emphasizes the importance of treating people equally. This idea perfectly matches the public health approach to alcohol issues, which highlights the importance of population-level policies to control drinking—such as raising the price of alcohol or limiting alcohol advertising—rather than policies that could stigmatize individual drinkers (Bruun, 1971; Tigerstedt, 1999). The importance of the public health perspective in Sweden can be seen in the government's 1977 decision to shift the authority over Swedish alcohol policy from the Ministry of Finance to the Ministry of Health and Social Affairs (Holder et al., 2008, p. 51)—a move firmly signaling the pre-eminence of public health concerns over economic concerns on the issue of alcohol.

The public health perspective has great salience not just in Sweden, but in the other Nordic countries as well. Interestingly, like Sweden, these countries have also typically maintained more restrictive alcohol policies than other European nations (Babor, 2004). For example, the Nordic countries helped facilitate the design and adoption of the European Commission's 2006 alcohol strategy (National Institute for Health and Welfare, 2012). Even the idea of, and the term, "alcohol policy"— which, as described in Chapter 1, is now used prominently in the literature—was first employed in the Nordic countries (Room, 1999). Given Chapter 4's discussion of the importance of history and culture, the impact of this legacy of strict policies and culture of public health ideas should not be underestimated—and needs to be considered when exploring the specific case study of Swedish policy change in the next section.

Case Study

The specific case study explored here is the way in which European Union (EU) membership affected Sweden's strict alcohol laws. Following a national referendum in November 1994, Sweden joined the EU on January 1, 1995 (Gustavsson, 2007). Given that one of the EU's aims is to encourage free movement of people and goods across member states' borders, a central issue in discussions about Sweden's accession was the fate of its restrictive alcohol laws. How could Sweden limit alcohol imports from countries with lower alcohol taxes and yet still remain faithful to the EU's founding principles?

The European Court of Justice was forced to consider this question, ruling that Sweden's restrictions on the amount of alcohol individuals could bring into Sweden from other EU countries were incompatible with the EU's common market philosophy (Bilefsky, 2007). Therefore, import quotas for individuals were harmonized with EU norms in 2004 ("Swedish alcohol intake ...", 2012). Additionally, Sweden was also forced to relinquish its monopoly over alcohol production and the *wholesale* selling of alcohol, although all other retail sales remained controlled by the Systembolaget (Nycander, 1998).

Despite the Court's ruling, concern that the Systembolaget might be dismantled by the EU remained high. In what was widely interpreted as an effort to ensure Sweden's retail monopoly was retained, in 2005 the Systembolaget launched a print and internet advertising campaign across Europe showing the social harms of alcohol and the importance of limiting excessive consumption (Bevanger, 2005). Concerns were also raised that the relaxation of import restrictions mandated by the Court might make it easier for teenagers—who were unable to purchase alcohol from an official Systembolaget shop—to obtain imported alcohol (Svensson, 2012).

Anxiety about imports undermining the Systembolaget prompted debates in Sweden about whether the government should cut alcohol taxes. Some commentary cited Finland's decision to lower its alcohol taxes in 2004 in an attempt to decrease individual imports from the neighboring EU country of Estonia, suggesting that, if alcohol taxes in Sweden were lower, the incentive for Swedes to purchase alcohol abroad would be reduced ("Sweden may cut ...", 2004). The effects of imported alcohol on overall consumption in Sweden were important to consider since, even in 2003 before Swedish import quotas fully harmonized with EU norms, 20 percent of the alcohol consumed in Sweden was purchased in Denmark (Lyall, 2003). Sweden's move to fully align its import restrictions with EU guidelines in 2004 came just months after Denmark had lowered its tax on spirits by nearly a half—prompting fears that Swedish travelers would flood their home country with these imports and substantially increase alcohol's social harms (see discussion in Gustafsson and Ramstedt, 2011, p. 433; Lyall, 2003). However, a time series analysis of the 2000–2007 period has suggested that not all of these fears came to fruition. Specifically, the study showed that rates of assault and alcohol-impaired driving in southern Sweden (the region of the country that is closest to Denmark) did not increase following the 2004 policy change, although acute alcohol poisonings did rise—particularly among individuals in their 50s and 60s (Gustafsson and Ramstedt, 2011). Another study that compared the fates of northern and southern Sweden also concluded that "the overall rates of reported alcohol-related problems in the southern and northern parts of Sweden did not change, ... although changes were observed in some population groups" (Gustafsson, 2010, p. 464).

Additionally, although per capita alcohol consumption in Sweden rose by 30 percent between 1995 (when Sweden formally joined the EU) and 2004, during the mid 2000s this increase halted despite the policy change that took place in 2004 (Andréasson, Nilsson, and Bränström, 2009). Nevertheless, adopting a more long-term view, data from a Swedish Board of Agriculture report indicates that alcohol consumption—particularly of beer and wine—rose more than *50 percent* in Sweden between 1995 and 2009, an increase the Board linked to the relaxation of import restrictions ("Swedish alcohol intake ...", 2012). These different figures indicate the difficulties of generalizing about the outcomes of alcohol policies, or assuming that such policies' effects will be predictable or straightforward.

Cross-Case Comparison

Comparing the Swedish case study to the case study of the Soviet Union discussed in the previous chapter is instructive. The Soviet Union case study showed how internal pressures—namely, a lack of public support and a loss of government revenue—significantly impeded the success of Gorbachev's effort to sharply reduce alcohol consumption in Soviet society (Herlihy, 2002). In Sweden, however, an external factor rather than internal pressure was ultimately responsible for the relaxation of its restrictive policies. Indeed, in contrast to the Soviet Union, Sweden's restrictive policies have traditionally enjoyed significant public support. Recent opinion polls indicate that such support remains prevalent, with one 2006 Systembolaget poll finding that 57 percent of respondents supported the alcohol retail monopoly (Holder et al., 2008, p. 15). Another set of polls found that Swedish attitudes toward alcohol policy actually became *slightly more restrictive* between 1995 and 2003, with most respondents favoring population-wide control measures in both periods (Hübner, 2012). Public support for such policies in Sweden is important, since, as previously discussed, public opinion can play a fundamental role in alcohol policymaking; more specifically, public support can be particularly important in ensuring that government alcohol monopolies remain workable (Kortteinen, 1989).

Globalization and Local Cultural Contexts

Yet public opinion alone does not determine alcohol policy. Sweden's experience shows that *external* pressures—in this case, the requirements of EU membership—can be just as influential as internal pressures like public opinion in shaping alcohol policies. The Swedish case study therefore supports Dobbin and colleagues' (2007) idea, discussed in Chapter 3, that encouragement and coercion by international organizations can be a key driver of policy diffusion.

The Swedish case study also supports the assertion made in Chapter 4 that, in recent times, European countries' alcohol policies have increasingly converged, turning away from policies that aim to restrict imports, changes that have been indirectly encouraged by the European Union's emphasis on free trade across internal European borders (Ahlström et al., 2004; Crawford and Tanner, 1995; National Institute for Health and Welfare, 2012). Of course, European alcohol policies are still not identical—some countries, such as the Nordic countries (including Sweden), maintain higher excise duties on alcohol than others (Babor, 2004). Nevertheless, the increasing convergence of such policies is an important development.

This convergence forces observers to confront an issue explored in Chapter 4: the distinct cultural norms present in different societies. Such distinct norms shape drinking practices and influence the scale of social harms associated with alcohol consumption (Gladwell, 2010; Heath, 1958). In Europe in particular, commentators have cited the difference between more regular and moderate drinking patterns in southern countries such as France and Italy, and more inconsistent and binge-oriented drinking patterns in northern countries such as the UK or Sweden (Engs, 1995). As discussed in Chapter 4, Österberg and Karlsson (2002, p. 18) have additionally noted that many northern countries lack the informal norms encouraging moderate consumption present in many southern countries; instead, these northern countries have developed stricter formal regulations to reduce excessive consumption. The case study of Sweden explored in this chapter raises the question of whether similar alcohol policies can work in very different drinking cultures. Sweden's "tradition of drinking to the point of drunkenness" (Daley, 2001, p. A1) has long been noted by observers (e.g., Lyall, 2003; "Loosening up ...", 2001). Yet the restrictive policies that have been developed in Sweden to reduce the social harms associated with these tendencies have, to a degree, been eroded by European integration. Can similar alcohol policies really accommodate both Italy and Sweden?

Dolowitz and Marsh's (2000) research has revealed that what "works" in one society does not always work when migrated elsewhere, even with modifications. One cannot expect that a policy that developed in one culture or country can be transferred unchanged to another culture or country. Even in the realm of alcohol policy, alcohol monopoly policies typically reflect different societies' specific cultures, political systems, and even religions (Babor, 2002; Kortteinen, 1989). Respecting these particularities can be difficult when alcohol policymaking is itself influenced by macro-level political, economic, and other forces. Ultimately the Swedish case study underlines the deep connections between alcohol policymaking and other kinds of policy decisions. The country's choice to pursue EU membership impacted the alcohol restrictions that its government was able to impose. Sometimes the influence of political and other factors can therefore limit the ability of alcohol policies to accommodate specific local needs and characteristics.

It is interesting to note that even countries that are not part of the EU have been affected by EU pressures and policy trends. Nordlund (2007), for example, has revealed how European integration has affected Norway's alcohol policies—even though Norway is not formally part of the EU. Specifically, Norway has felt many of the same pressures to loosen restrictions on alcohol imports that Sweden also experienced. The fact that a country that is not part of the EU can still be affected by its policy changes illustrates the far-reaching influence of such macro-level political, economic, and other forces.

Finally, it is important to note that although the Swedish case study focused on free movement of goods across borders, this is no longer the EU chief or sole priority on the issue of alcohol policymaking. In recent years, public health concerns have also become increasingly important in EU alcohol policymaking (National Institute for Health and Welfare, 2012). For example, as discussed in Chapter 4, the European Commission's 2006 alcohol strategy emphasizes the importance of reducing underage drinking, prenatal exposure to alcohol, and other public health-related harms (*European strategy* ..., 2011). Additionally, since 1999, within the European Commission the Directorate-General for Health and Consumer Protection (DG SANCO) has maintained authority over issues related to alcohol and health (Örnberg, 2013)—a further sign that alcohol is *not* only seen in an economic light within the EU.

Future Predictions

Despite the European Court of Justice's ruling in the 1990s, the Systembolaget's long-term future remains a subject of debate within Sweden. In particular, a further 2007 ruling by the Court paved the way for Swedish citizens to purchase alcohol from other European countries over the internet, further undermining the Systembolaget's monopoly (Bilefsky, 2007). Indeed, a year after that legal decision, the Systembolaget sold less than half of all alcohol consumed in Sweden, leading commentators to question whether it could still be called a "monopoly" at all (Majzner, 2008).

   In addition to the challenge of predicting what will happen to the Systembolaget, it is also difficult to guess what the *effects* of Sweden's significant alcohol policy changes will be. Estimating the effects of policy changes on alcohol consumption levels presents extraordinary methodological challenges (see, e.g., Gustafsson and Ramstedt, 2011). The challenges—and complex findings—of research into the effects of alcohol policy liberalization in the 1990s and 2000s were discussed earlier in this chapter. Predictive research is even more difficult to undertake; however, a 2010 study by Norström and colleagues projected that, in Sweden, replacing the alcohol monopoly with private stores would lead to a 17 percent increase in alcohol consumption, as well as more than 8,000 additional assaults each year. This matches the assertion that more comprehensive state monopolies are typically associated with lower rates of per capita alcohol consumption (Kortteinen, 1989; see also discussion in Babor, 2002). Ultimately the uncertainty surrounding future policy decisions and those decisions' effects means that, in the coming years, Sweden will continue to be a fascinating case study.

Case Study: Rounds and Pints in the UK

Many of the themes discussed in the previous section are also relevant to the next two case studies discussed in this chapter: the British traditions of drinking in rounds, and of drinking beer in pint measurements. Specifically, these two case studies also underline the importance of cultural and historical factors in shaping drinking patterns and attitudes toward alcohol. The alcohol policies discussed within these case studies, however, are very different from the restrictive policies examined in the previous Swedish case study. Indeed, the policies discussed do not mandate or restrict behavior; instead, they encourage—or "nudge"—individuals to make harm-minimizing choices.

These policies can therefore be seen as examples of nudge theory—a framework for influencing human behavior without emphasizing formal bans and increased restrictions that has been promoted in recent years by the economist Richard Thaler and the legal scholar Cass Sunstein (McSmith, 2010; Sugden, 2009). Thaler and Sunstein (2008, p. 6) have formally defined a nudge as "any aspect of the choice architecture that alters people's behavior in a predictable way without forbidding any options or significantly changing their economic incentives." Examples of nudges would include highlighting key points in government letters to citizens or making pension/retirement savings plans opt-out rather than opt-in systems.

The simplicity and unrestrictive nature of nudge theory has increased its appeal among politicians. In the UK, for example, after the Conservative–Liberal Democrat coalition government was formed in 2010, the Cabinet Office began eight "nudge theory" trials; specifically, these trials tested whether small changes, such as alterations to the language used in government documents, could lead to increased tax compliance and other outcomes desired by the government ("Nudge theory trials ...", 2012). The trials produced encouraging initial results. A Behavioural Insight Team—dubbed a "nudge unit" in *The Guardian*—was even set up within the Cabinet Office, and looked to Richard Thaler for advice (Wintour, 2010).

Of course, nudge theory has its critics and, like all theories, has limitations. In particular, questions have been raised about whether nudges alone can tackle complex public health-related social harms such as obesity—or, one might add, alcohol misuse ("Nudge theory trials ...", 2012). One official from the Department of Health, for example, told the House of Lords' science and technology committee: "There are not any silver bullets. While nudge is very useful, there are a whole range of interventions necessary to create behaviour change" (as quoted in "Nudge theory of social change ...", 2010).

Despite nudge theory's obvious limitations, its ostensible influence over some recent UK policy decisions represents a significant development in the application of theory and research to policymaking. Indeed, its influence offers some support for Weiss' (1982; 1999) ideas about the impact of research evidence. As described in detail in Chapter 3, Weiss has posited that although the findings of one particular study are unlikely to affect policy, the *general ideas* that emerge from a field can influence discourse. In this case nudge theory's *general* ideas— and the overall empirical conclusions of research undertaken by Thaler, Sunstein, and others in this area—seem to have had an impact. The question of whether and how such ideas might influence alcohol policy is the subject of the case studies described below.

Drinking in Rounds

Drinking in rounds is a social practice in which each person in a group takes turns buying a drink for everyone else in the group as well as themselves. This tradition has a long history in the UK; it was first described in the Oxford English

Dictionary as early as 1633 (Rohrer, 2008). In addition to the UK, drinking in rounds is also an ingrained cultural practice in Ireland, Australia, and New Zealand, all countries with historical links to Britain. The practice highlights how alcohol consumption can have profound social connotations. As Pernanen (2001, p. 57) has explained: "Rounds are bought to symbolize common bonds and obligations to the group." Drinking in rounds can reinforce friendships and strengthen group solidarity. Among previous generations, the practice was traditionally undertaken by groups of working-class men, helping to cement male friendships and build trust (Heath, 1995; Jayne, Valentine, and Holloway, 2010, p. 17). These gender- and class-based facets further underline the importance of historical and cultural factors in understanding drinking patterns.

Recently, however, drinking in rounds has been criticized by some experts who worry it might facilitate excessive consumption by forcing slower drinkers to consume drinks as quickly as the fastest drinker in the group (O'Neill, 2006). The Shropshire NHS Trust (2011), for example, advises that individuals can reduce their drinking "by opting for smaller rounds with only a couple of friends within your group or giving rounds a miss." Most notably, Richard Thaler, the proponent of nudge theory, has suggested that drinking in rounds might boost consumption rates by making individuals feel socially obligated to consume and purchase more drinks than they would consume otherwise (Hope, 2011). Instead, Thaler has recommended that groups of three or more should abandon the tradition of drinking in rounds and request a joint tab. Switching from round-based drinking to tab-based drinking can thus be seen as a potential "nudge" measure to reduce excessive drinking.

Interestingly, the criticisms advanced by Thaler and other experts do not represent the first critique of the drinking-in-rounds tradition. During WWI, buying rounds of drinks was banned in certain areas as the excessive consumption that accompanied it was believed to be hindering the war effort (de Castella, 2012). Such criticisms are not unique to the UK either. Concerns have also been raised in Ireland, where one 2006 news bulletin warned that people might inadvertently binge drink if a large number of people were included in the round (McConnell, 2006). The same report also cited the health minister for the Opposition as saying that although eschewing round-based drinking might be seen as antisocial, such a move *would* reduce alcohol's social harms. Similarly, in 2006 the Scottish Executive also expressed concern that the tradition of drinking in rounds was detrimental to public health (Coughlan, 2006). The NHS for Greater Glasgow and Clyde (2012) recommends "drinking water every second or alternative drink" or simply opting "out of rounds altogether" to reduce one's consumption.

Yet these criticisms of the tradition—and Thaler's recommendations in particular—have prompted some debate among commentators. Much of this debate has been deliberately tongue-in-cheek, but has highlighted the long history and ingrained cultural nature of the practice. For example, one commentator wrote in *The Telegraph* that "only an American" would make such a suggestion about abandoning this British tradition and that "Thaler will find most pub-goers would rather risk binge-drinking than being deemed tight-fisted" (Pelling, 2011). These and similar comments illustrate the very serious point that cultural practices, however damaging to public health, can be difficult to overcome.

As of the time of writing, the suggestion not to drink in rounds remains just that—a suggestion promoted by some NHS trusts. In this sense, the official cautions issued about round-based drinking do not yet constitute a policy change. However, a second case study—drinking beer in pint measures—*is* related to an actual recent policy change in the UK. Like drinking in rounds, drinking in pints also shows the importance of cultural and historical factors in shaping drinking patterns and attitudes toward alcohol policies.

Drinking in Pints

Drinking beer in pint measures also has a long history in Britain, almost as long as the history of drinking in rounds. Researchers commonly date the practice to a 1698 Act of Parliament which mandated that beer could only be sold in pints or multiples of pint measures (e.g., quarts) (Cole, 2011). Today beer is still typically served in pints and half-pints in the UK, with alcohol servers ensuring these precise measurements are met. Indeed, it is illegal for pubs to give short measures (The Royal Borough of Windsor and Maidenhead, 2012).

Selling beer in pint and half-pint measures offers drinkers some advantages. In particular it helps drinkers ensure that they receive their money's worth, and it facilitates drinkers' efforts to compare quality across pubs and bars. Yet this practice also has the potential to increase alcohol's social harms. Today many strong imported lagers are commonly consumed in pint measures in the UK, yet such high-alcohol beers were not originally meant to be consumed in such large quantities ("In praise of ...", 2011). Until recently, however, legislation has prevented servers from offering alternative measures (beyond pints, half-pints, and thirds of pints) that might better suit these higher-strength drinks (Associated Press, 2011).

In January 2011, however, the UK government announced that pubs and bars in Britain would be allowed to sell beer in measures equivalent to *two-thirds* of a pint, a measure commonly termed a schooner (additionally, such establishments would also be allowed to sell measures of wine less than 75ml) ("Schooner set ...", 2011). The government primarily framed this decision as an effort to cut "red tape" and offer businesses more freedom, rather than as an effort to promote public health. Specifically, the government's science minister said: "We are freeing businesses so they can innovate and create new products to meet the demands of their customers" (as quoted in Smithers, 2011). Some representatives from the pub industry welcomed the change; the chief executive of the Beer and Pub Association, for example, praised the "greater flexibility" that the new policy allowed (as quoted in "Schooners to be served ...", 2011). Most relevantly, the chief executive of an alcohol awareness organization highlighted an additional potential benefit of the new policy: it could encourage people to drink smaller amounts of alcohol (Smithers, 2011).

Offering two-thirds of a pint is a nudge policy, according to Thaler and Sunstein's (2008) definition as it changes the alternatives available to drinkers in a way that might encourage them to drink less—but does not restrict their alternatives. By emphasizing minor, non-invasive policy changes, nudge theory shares similarities with "policy incrementalism," the framework advanced by Lindblom (1959; 1979) that was discussed in detail in Chapter 3, and is one of the most influential frameworks in political science. This framework posits that policymaking typically consists of small, incremental changes rather than dramatic shifts, and policy change is thus more of an incremental than revolutionary process. Such small changes could include nudges.

As with drinking in rounds, not all public reactions to this policy change were wholly positive, however. For example, a spokesperson for the Campaign for Real Ale (CAMRA), an organization that promotes real ale and local pubs, cautioned that it was still unknown "whether such a new measure will benefit drinkers or simply cause confusion," and observed that stocking this different size of glasses could prove costly for pubs (as quoted in Hall, 2011). An article in the UK national newspaper the *Mirror* described the change this way: "Two-thirds of a pint of lager and a packet of crisps please, barman. It may sound odd but this is what drinkers will soon be able to order after one of the biggest changes to booze measures for more than 300 years" (Manning, 2011).

This idea that a request for two-thirds of a pint "sound[s] odd" shows the difficulty of overcoming ingrained historical and cultural traditions—even when these traditions were, like drinking in pints, created by historical government policy and in spite of the potential associated harms. Indeed, when considering both the drinking-in-rounds and the drinking-in-pints case studies it is important to remember that, just as drinking patterns are influenced by historical and cultural factors, attitudes toward drinking are shaped by these same forces. For example, Nicholls (2010) has showed how concerns about excessive alcohol consumption have emerged during numerous, *particular* historical moments in the British past. Nicholls' work illustrates that such concerns cannot be fully understood without probing the political and social contexts in which they arose, and that debates about alcohol issues have typically reflected larger societal concerns about the extent of individual freedom and the proper role of markets in a liberal society. Nicholls has described how, in the period following the Restoration of the monarchy in the seventeenth century, one's wine, beer, and port choices helped signify political party allegiance—an important act in a period of intense partisan politics (p. 52). Today's political and ideological climate, where enthusiasm for free markets and suspicion of restricting access to alcohol are prominent, has likely increased the appeal of using non-mandate-based approaches to tackle alcohol's social harms. Nudges such as alternatives to drinking in rounds and serving alcohol in a variety of measures fit in well with this political and ideological climate, as well as with a public opinion that typically favors less invasive strategies that do not restrict the availability of alcohol (Giesbrecht et al., 2007; Greenfield et al., 2007).

Conclusion

At first glance, the alcohol policies examined in the Swedish and British case studies presented in this chapter could not be more different. The government-controlled monopoly system examined in the Swedish case study constitutes a comprehensive approach to reducing alcohol consumption and its related social harms, whilst the "nudge" suggestions in the British case study are less rigid and less comprehensive policy suggestions. Yet these two examples both illustrate the importance of history, culture, and public opinion in designing alcohol policies. Nowhere is it easy to move against the grain of long-held traditional practices—especially when such practices, such as the monopoly system in Sweden and drinking in rounds in the UK, seem to enjoy public support (Holder et al., 2008, p. 15; Pelling, 2011). Even when domestic governments or supranational organizations—such as the EU in the case of Sweden—spearhead initiatives that move against cultural traditions, implementing such initiatives can constitute a significant challenge. To offer one further example of this, although public opinion generally favors the monopoly system in Sweden (Holder et al., 2008, p. 15), it is almost impossible to imagine such a system being successfully installed in the UK in the near future. The lack of a history of such a system and the UK's different cultural attitudes to alcohol— illustrated by the criticisms that greeted even the nudge policy decisions—mean that any effort to implement such a system there would likely be undermined, much like Gorbachev's anti-alcohol campaign in the Soviet Union.

One final theme from this chapter that merits discussion is the presence of intriguing parallels between the Swedish case study and that of the Oglala Sioux Nation's Pine Ridge Reservation, which was described in Chapter 1. The Oglala Sioux's prohibition policy was undermined by the rampant availability of alcohol in the nearby town of Whiteclay—outside of tribal control (Williams, 2012)—and, as a result, alcohol misuse remains a significant problem in Pine Ridge. Sweden has similarly been affected by the decisions of other European countries to sell alcohol at lower prices, and by the EU's policy of emphasizing free trade. These decisions have undermined Sweden's ability to impose its own alcohol regulations and restrict the supply of alcohol within its borders. Of course, Sweden's case differs sharply from that of the Oglala Sioux because Sweden actively decided to seek EU membership. Despite this important distinction, though, both case studies illustrate the challenges societies face when they endeavor to maintain unique alcohol policies in an interconnected world. Indeed, as discussed in Chapter 3, improved technology, better transportation, and heightened globalization have led to an *internationalization* of alcohol issues—and this trend is likely to continue in coming decades. As discussed in Chapter 1, some public health experts have argued that such internationalization means that alcohol's social harms can only be effectively tackled through an international approach. The WHO, for example, has endeavored to promote an international approach to alcohol's social harms. This chapter's case studies serve as telling reminders of a tension between the international nature of alcohol issues and the need to navigate, and be sensitive to, local historical and cultural factors.

Chapter 7
Targeted Policies:
Minimum Drinking Age Laws

The aim of most of the policy efforts described in the previous chapters—such as government alcohol retail monopolies, prohibition campaigns, advisories not to drink in rounds—was to reduce consumption in general, or decrease alcohol's *overall* social harms. Yet more targeted alcohol policies that focus on *particular* social harms have also been implemented in many countries. This chapter explores such policies, and whether the factors that influence their adoption differ from the factors that influence the adoption of more general alcohol policies, and also further tests the explanatory value of the ideas put forward in chapters 3 and 4, such as the importance of history and culture in alcohol policy and the key role often played by interest groups.

Targeted policies include measures such as warning labels on alcoholic beverages to reduce fetal alcohol syndrome, or stricter blood-alcohol limits to reduce alcohol-involved driving. The three case studies examined in detail in this chapter, however, all consist of changes in the minimum drinking age, or the minimum age at which individuals can purchase or consume alcohol. Such changes can be seen as targeted policies as their intention is to specifically reduce the social harms of alcohol use among young people. In particular, by adopting the first two policies examined here—the implementation of higher minimum drinking ages in both the US state of Michigan and then throughout the US—policymakers aimed to reduce alcohol-involved traffic accidents among the 18-to-20 age group (Voas and Fell, 2010). The third case study explored in this chapter focuses on an inverse strategy: the decision in New Zealand to *lower* the minimum age required to purchase alcohol from 20 years to 18 years (Wanberg, Timken, and Milkman, 2010, p. 117). The differences and similarities among the US and New Zealand policy experiences are probed in detail.

All three case studies illustrate the role that evidence—and, more broadly, beliefs about the policies' effectiveness—can play in the adoption of alcohol policies. The national policy change in the US has been cited by scholars as a hopeful example of how research *can* play a role in alcohol policymaking (Toomey and Rosenfeld, 1996; Voas and Fell, 2010, p. 17). Evidence also played a role in policy debates in both Michigan and New Zealand, as is illustrated in the analysis later in this chapter. Despite evidence's prominence, however, the three case studies do not wholly validate Lasswell's (1951) optimistic vision of policy-oriented research, outlined in Chapter 3—nor do the case studies solely refute the pessimistic "two communities" perspective (Caplan, 1979; Rich, 1991,

p. 324). Instead, as this chapter shows, the case studies tell more complex stories about how policymakers interpret research evidence, and the factors that can constrain the role of research in policymakers' decisions. In particular, the case studies reinforce the idea that evidence does not influence policy in a vacuum; many other forces, such as pressure from the public and interest groups, as well as more practical concerns, are also often at the forefront of policymakers' minds.

Historical Background

At the heart of all three case studies is the issue of youth drinking, and whether alcohol consumption should be reserved for those individuals over a certain age. Interestingly, Warner's (1998) study of drinking norms in pre-industrial England has revealed that separate drinking standards for adults and juveniles were only promoted after 1500; prior to this date, in the late medieval period, both adults and juveniles were similarly advised to engage only in moderate alcohol consumption. The idea that juveniles should be abstinent—a notion central to many minimum drinking age laws established in the twentieth century—was not prominent in the discourse. According to Warner's analysis, specific concerns about juveniles gaining access to alcohol did not gain salience until the 1540s.

In the US, beginning in the 1880s, some states instituted policies limiting minors' ability to purchase or consume alcoholic beverages (Rosenthal, 1988, p. 652; Treuthart, 2005, p. 106). By the early twentieth century, youth drinking began to receive greater attention in American society, as shown by the emergence of studies and news reports examining this issue. In 1935, for example, a survey of thousands of American youths found that a majority of boys and more than two-fifths of girls under the age of 21 drank alcohol—results that were published in *Life* magazine (Bell, 1938; see also "Youth tell their story ...", 1938, p. 20). This study and others like it not only reveal the prevalence of youth drinking in previous generations, but also illustrate that *concern* about such drinking is not solely a twenty-first-century phenomenon.

Today many countries have implemented minimum drinking ages, although the specific content of these laws varies widely. For example, Italy maintains no minimum age for private consumption, but enforces a minimum age of 16 for *public* consumption of alcohol; in Greece, one must be at least 17 to purchase alcohol, but one can consume alcohol at 14 (Hasin and Keyes, 2011, p. 33). Thus, although the case studies of Michigan, the US, and New Zealand are the focus of this chapter, the issue of minimum drinking ages—and how to best design related policies—has wider relevance.

Problem Scope

A key aim of the US minimum drinking age policies that were instituted in the late 1970s and 1980s was to reduce alcohol-involved traffic accidents among young people (Cook and Gearing, 2012, p. 277; Voas and Fell, 2010). Such accidents constitute one of alcohol's most substantial and pressing social harms. Even today motor vehicle accidents remain a significant cause of death for young adults in many developed countries—and alcohol often plays a role in such tragedies. In the US, for example, 22 percent of drivers aged 16–20 involved in fatal accidents in 2004 were under the influence of alcohol (National Highway Traffic Safety Administration, 2006). Researchers from the Centers for Disease Control and Prevention (CDC) have estimated that, in 2010, nearly 11,000 people in the US died as a result of alcohol-involved traffic accidents (Bergen, Shults, and Rudd, 2011). In the European Union, alcohol plays a role in more than 17,000 traffic fatalities each year, according to the Institute of Alcohol Studies (Anderson, 2008, p. 8).

The case studies below illustrate that reducing such accidents was a primary driver of the US minimum age policies, yet such accidents are not the only social harm that can be reduced through instituting minimum drinking ages. For example, some research has also found a minimum age of 21 to be associated with reductions in youth suicide (Birckmayer and Hemenway, 1999) and reductions in arrests for vandalism and disorderly conduct (Joksch and Jones,1993). More generally, in a thorough review of high-quality previous research, Wagenaar and Toomey (2002) found that a third of the studies they uncovered that examined the effects of minimum drinking age policies found that these policies were associated with lower levels of overall drinking; only one study indicated the opposite relationship—that a minimum age policy was associated with higher levels of drinking. These potential additional policy effects—beyond reductions in alcohol-involved traffic accidents among young people—are important to keep in mind when exploring the American case studies in the next few sections.

Case Study: National Level in the US

When Prohibition ended in 1933, many US states enacted legislation setting a minimum drinking age of 21 years; however, in the 1970s some of these states began to lower their minimum ages to 20, 19, or, most prominently, 18 (Cook and Gearing, 2010). This trend towards lowering the minimum age during the 1970s was prompted by the passage of the Twenty-sixth Amendment to the US Constitution in 1971; the Amendment lowered the minimum voting age from 21 to 18 and was itself prompted in part by the Vietnam War draft, in which men as young as 18 were conscripted (Deloria and Wilkins, 1999, p. 154; Legge, 1991). Many policymakers reasoned that if individuals could vote and be drafted into the armed forces at age 18, they should be given the full rights of adulthood at age 18 as well, including the right to purchase or consume alcohol (Williams, 2011). Once some states lowered their drinking ages, residents of other states occasionally expressed concerns that, if their state did not follow suit, then teenagers would simply drive across the state border to purchase alcohol—thus raising the risk of alcohol-involved traffic accidents (Legge, 1991). Some states' efforts to lower their drinking ages therefore prompted other states to make the same policy change, a clear example of policy diffusion, the phenomenon described in Chapter 3 (Berry and Berry, 1990).

Motivating Factors

By the early 1980s, however, concern about alcohol's social harms—and, in particular, the harm of alcohol-involved traffic accidents among young people—had increased. The sources for this increased concern were multifold and included research studies which showed that some states' decisions to *lower* their drinking ages were associated with *higher* rates of alcohol-related traffic deaths among the 18-to-20 age group (Cook and Tauchen, 1984), or that states' decisions to *raise* their drinking ages were associated with *lower* rates of such deaths in the affected age group (Williams et al., 1983). Additionally Hingson and colleagues (1984) found that a higher drinking age was associated with a lower frequency of driving after consuming alcohol among teenagers. In 1982, the National Transportation Safety Board, a federal government agency, publicly emphasized the link between alcohol consumption and traffic fatalities among young drivers (Mittelman, 2008, p. 175). This instance of research evidence's role in raising awareness and motivating policy action is a noteworthy phenomenon, and is analyzed in more detail in the next section of this chapter.

A second factor behind the increased concern about alcohol-involved traffic accidents during the 1980s was a campaign by committed pressure groups, such as Mothers Against Drunk Drinking (MADD), to raise awareness of the potentially tragic consequences of alcohol-impaired driving. Candy Lightner founded MADD in 1980 after her teenage daughter was killed by a drunk driver; at a national press conference on Capitol Hill in Washington, DC, later in 1980, she brought substantial public attention to this issue (Davies, 2005). In 1983, a TV movie about MADD aired on the national network NBC raising further awareness of the cause ("MADD milestones", 2005). During the 1980s, MADD's influence spread through the founding of hundreds of local groups across the US; a second national organization, Remove Intoxicated Drivers (RID), which focused on similar concerns, also gained prominence during this period (McCarthy and Wolfson, 1996).

MADD's efforts to give a voice to victims and victims' families helped both policymakers and the general public become more aware of the potential harms of alcohol-impaired driving (Voas and Fell, 2010). Indeed, as Treuthart (2005, pp. 108–9) has observed, once the issue of a minimum drinking age began to be debated in Congress, "MADD continued an active advocacy role and spurred on the rhetoric utilized by the bill's supporters by centering it on drunk driving victims and their families." The influence of MADD and other organized groups on this issue offers support for Weiss' (1983) idea that competing interests shape policymaking and reveals that such interests are not solely driven by economic imperatives; they can also be led by ordinary citizens and driven by social concerns. This sense that the general public demanded action was encapsulated by President Ronald Reagan's statement in late 1982 that the American public wanted "the slaughter on the highways to stop" (as quoted in Mittelman, 2008, p. 175). Like the temperance groups that facilitated the adoption of Prohibition in the early-twentieth-century, the role of MADD and similar groups in promoting anti-drunk driving policies highlights the continuing significance of popular activism in this area (Schrad, 2010).

A third factor that contributed to increased concern about alcohol during the 1980s was the political climate and the growing prominence of fears about illegal drugs. This decade witnessed the escalation of the "crack epidemic" and the passage of several national laws that aimed to reduce and deter drug-involved offending. During this same period Reagan's White House sometimes framed alcohol as a "gateway drug" that would lead drinkers to consume illegal substances (Mendelson, 2009, p. 164). The intensifying "drug war" and the link between alcohol abuse and the abuse of illegal drugs likely helped foment a political climate sympathetic to establishing a national minimum age. Such a sympathetic political climate likely was a key step in the policy's eventual adoption, since Kingdon's (2003) theory of agenda-setting—discussed in Chapter 3—posits that such a climate is necessary for a policy to rise onto the legislative agenda.

A final important factor motivating legislative action was the choice of several US states to impose higher minimum drinking ages *before* the federal policy was adopted. Indeed, "by the end of 1980, fourteen of the thirty states that had lowered their drinking ages ... had raised them, although not necessarily back to the original limits" (Williams et al., 1983, p. 169). By 1983, 16 states had reinstated a minimum age of 21 (MADD, 2012). Although, in the US, the relationship between state governments' legislative decisions and the federal government's legislative decisions can be complex (Welch and Thompson, 1980), federal policymakers must have been aware of states' choices and such choices likely further underlined the salience of this issue. The Michigan case study explored later in this chapter offers insight into states' decisions to change their minimum age policies.

Federal action began to be taken in 1983 when the Presidential Commission on Drunk Driving—which counted Candy Lightner, the founder of MADD, as well as the president of the brewing industry's trade association among its members— posited that the federal government should set a minimum drinking age of 21 by denying states federal money for highways if they did not adopt this policy (Mittelman, 2008). The fact that the president of the brewing industry's trade association was a member of this commission is important to note, as it signals that the industry was certainly not uniformly and staunchly opposed to the policy. Additionally, members of Congress argued that instituting a nationwide minimum age of 21 would save lives—perhaps 730 each year (as cited in Mendelson, 2009,

p. 166 and Males, 1986, p. 181). The prevalence of this straightforward and salient statistic in the national debate highlights how certain research findings can gain significant influence in the policymaking process, an issue discussed in more detail later in this chapter.

In its 1984 National Minimum Drinking Age Act, the federal government did indeed institute a national minimum age of 21 for the purchase and public possession of alcohol; states which did not raise their minimum age to 21 risked forfeiting federal funding for their highways (Williams, 2011). The bill was sponsored by a Democratic senator but signed into law by the Republican President Ronald Reagan, and, ultimately, "less than a handful of members of Congress" actively opposed the bill, indicating the extensive—and bipartisan—support it received (Lerner, 2011, p. 90; Treuthart, 2005, p. 110).

After the law's passage, many states, concerned about losing highway funding, promptly raised their minimum ages (Robin, 1991, p. 113). The state of South Dakota challenged the constitutionality of the federal law, arguing that the authority of states to set their own alcohol policies, such as minimum drinking age policies, was enshrined in the Constitution's Twenty-first Amendment, which had ended Prohibition (Uradnik, 2011, p. 171). The resultant legal case, *South Dakota v. Dole*, was argued before the US Supreme Court in 1987. The Supreme Court upheld the federal legislation, endorsing the federal government's power to use its taxing and spending powers to promote a public health issue (Stephens and Scheb, 2012, p. 165). The key element of this controversy was the exercise of federal power, rather than objections to a minimum drinking age in principle (Coleman, 1984; Temkin and Roelke, 2009, p. 231). This nuance is important as it shows that the issue of an alcohol policy may itself not necessarily be controversial—rather the way in which a policy is advanced can provoke resistance.

The court challenge offers several important similarities with the Swedish example of import quotas, discussed in detail in Chapter 6. As in Sweden, where the EU played an important supranational role in relaxing such quotas in the 1990s and early 2000s (Bilefsky, 2007; Nycander, 1998), the federal government exerted significant influence over many states' decisions to increase their drinking ages to 21. In both examples, such policy changes were prompted by the possibility of serious consequences for noncompliance; in Sweden the ultimate sanction was loss of EU common market membership, and in the US the loss of essential highway funds. Dobbin and colleagues (2007) have discussed the way in which both encouragement and coercion by international organizations, such as the World Trade Organization (WTO), can drive policy diffusion. Although the EU and the national government in the US are not international organizations, these case studies show how they have used the same forces of encouragement and coercion to instigate policy change. Thus, even when considering alcohol policymaking at the more local level, it is essential not to forget the potential influence of Washington, Brussels, or other larger governmental entities. As these case studies illustrate, such external forces can be very powerful indeed.

Ultimately, despite South Dakota's court challenge, by 1988 all US states had established a minimum legal drinking age of 21, which applied to both the purchase and public consumption of alcohol (Fell et al., 2009; Uradnik, 2011).

Evidence

The example of the National Minimum Drinking Age Act deserves scrutiny because of the role that research evidence played in its passage. As described in the previous section, one factor that increased the national salience of this issue was a series of research studies produced during the early 1980s which suggested that some states' decisions to *lower* their drinking ages were associated with *higher* rates of alcohol-related traffic deaths among the 18-to-20 age group (Cook and Tauchen, 1984), or that states' decisions to *raise* their drinking ages were associated with *lower* rates of such deaths in the affected age group (Williams et al., 1983).

This prominent deployment of evidence in the policymaking process has led Voas and Fell (2010, p. 18) and Toomey and Rosenfeld (1996) to cite the federal minimum drinking age as a positive example of research evidence helping to shape alcohol policymaking. At first glance, the collaboration of the research and policy communities in this case study might therefore be seen as a tangible example of Lasswell's (1951) optimistic vision. The case study also purports to sharply challenge the "two communities" thesis, whereby researchers and policymakers are seen as fundamentally unable to work together (Caplan, 1979; Rich, 1991, p. 324). Yet this case study is not a straightforward "success" story, and its complexities reveal many of the challenges inherent in drives for evidence-based policymaking. First, as Wagenaar (1983a) identified at the time, some of the research highlighted by some stakeholder groups in debates about the effects of lowering the drinking age contained methodological limitations, raising questions about whether it should have been presented in support of the policy. It was also later claimed that, when debating the national legislation, policymakers relied too heavily on a single study that focused only on short-term impacts, thus magnifying the policy's potential positive consequences (as described in Treuthart, 2005, p. 110; Males, 1986, pp. 181–2). These criticisms are interesting, as they offer a real-life case study of the debates about presentation of evidence described in Chapter 3. Naturally, all research contains methodological limitations and nuanced findings that cannot be easily summarized. Yet, even when evidence does appear to influence policymaking, as in this example, the question remains as to whether that research is *rigorous* enough that it *should* influence policymaking.

Despite these controversies over evidence, it is clear that between 1988 and 1995, alcohol-involved traffic deaths among young people aged 15 to 20 fell by nearly a half (National Highway Traffic Safety Administration, 2007; also cited in Fell et al., 2009; Voas and Fell, 2010). Examining a longer timescale, the number of such deaths among young people aged 16 to 20 declined 62 percent between 1982 and 2008 (National Institute on Alcohol Abuse and Alcoholism, n.d.). In the mid 1970s, more than 60 percent of traffic deaths were alcohol-related;

by 2010 this statistic had reduced to just 31 percent (National Highway Traffic Safety Administration, 2011; National Institute on Alcohol Abuse and Alcoholism, n.d.). The question of whether these reductions in harm are directly related to the establishment of the minimum drinking age has received significant attention from researchers; indeed, the question is among the most-studied issues in alcohol policy scholarship. Although it is impossible in this chapter to explore the details of all of the studies that have examined this question, several key findings stand out.

It is clear that after a minimum drinking age of 21 was adopted in New York State, self-reported alcohol purchases by young people aged 19 and 20 fell by some 70 percent, and alcohol consumption among the same age group fell by up to a quarter (Yu, Varone, and Shacket, 1997). More pointedly, statistical analyses based on Wisconsin's experiences in the 1980s suggest that a higher minimum drinking age was linked to lower levels of alcohol-related traffic crashes among 18-, 19-, and 20-year-olds (Figlio, 1995).

This conclusion is borne out by several broader literature reviews. Wagenaar and Toomey's (2002) extensive review, for example, explored 79 rigorous analyses published between 1960 and 1999 that examined the relationship between the minimum drinking age and alcohol-related traffic accidents. More than half of these analyses found that increases in the minimum drinking age were associated with subsequent decreases in such accidents. After reviewing 49 empirical studies, Shults and colleagues (2001, p. 75) similarly concluded that "there is strong evidence that MLDA [minimum legal drinking age] laws, particularly those that set the MLDA at age 21, are effective in preventing alcohol-related crashes and associated injuries."

Yet, once again, the "story" told by research evidence is not entirely straightforward. One recent study by Miron and Tetelbaum (2009b) found that the adoption of the federal minimum drinking age of 21 was *not* associated with any overall reduction in teenage traffic fatalities. Unlike some previous studies in this area, the authors controlled for potentially confounding variables such as the adoption of lower speed limits in some states at the same time. Additionally, as was already discussed, many states had already raised their drinking ages *prior* to the adoption of national legislation—and, according to the study's authors, such state-level changes might have actually been responsible for the reductions in fatalities (Miron and Tetelbaum 2009a; 2009b). A further complicating issue is that, at the same time that they raised their minimum drinking age, many states also established zero-tolerance laws, which made it illegal for drivers under the age of 21 from driving with *any* alcohol in their systems. Separating the effects of higher minimum drinking ages from the effects of these zero-tolerance laws is exceedingly difficult (Voas, Tippetts, and Fell, 2003). Nevertheless, Voas and colleagues (2003), who raised this issue, still concluded that both policies were helping to reduce the proportion of fatal traffic accidents involving alcohol.

One final consequence of the policy change that also deserves consideration here is that 18-to-20-year-old drinkers became subject to new offenses; what had been perfectly legal activities—purchasing and consuming alcohol—were criminalized. This side effect has been examined by Wolfson and Hourigan (1997, p. 1161), who have argued that the imposition of the minimum age of 21 likely contributed to the increase in arrest rates among 18-to-20-year-olds that occurred in the US in the years after this policy's adoption. Since arrests can have serious repercussions for individuals' lives and career paths, the policy's consequences in this area should not be overlooked.

This brief summary of findings and impacts illustrates how difficult it must be for policymakers to sort through different studies' conflicting conclusions. Even for this single policy, which has already been described in this chapter as one of the most-researched alcohol policy changes in history, evaluations have not been unanimously positive in their findings. Such diversity illustrates yet another challenge of trying to engage in evidence-based policymaking.

Case Study: State-Level Policy Change in the US (Michigan)

The previous case study illustrated how the movement for a national minimum drinking age may have been encouraged by several states' decisions to reinstate a drinking age of 21. The case study in this section explores why one state decided to act before the federal government prompted it to do so. The US state of Michigan initially lowered its minimum drinking age from January 1, 1972, and then raised it again, first to 19 years on December 22, 1978, and then to 21 from January 1, 1979 (Begun, 1980). The causes and consequences of these policy changes are examined, as is the question of whether the circumstances and factors which motivated legislative action in Michigan also motivated later action at the national level. This dramatic period and its complex decisions has been explored in detail by Begun (1980), Legge (1991), Wagenaar (1993), and Toomey, Nelson, and Lenk (2009) and the discussion in the following two subsections analyzes the findings of this previous research, assessing whether the theories described in chapters 3 and 4 apply to this case study of US state-level alcohol policymaking.

Factors Motivating the Decrease

As described earlier in this chapter, after the Twenty-sixth Amendment—which reduced the national minimum *voting* age from 21 to 18—was adopted in 1971, many states, including Michigan, decided to similarly reduce their minimum drinking ages (Deloria and Wilkins, 1999, p. 154; Legge, 1991). Although some controversy greeted this policy decision in Michigan (Begun, 1980), advocates advanced several key arguments in favor of the change. According to Legge (1991), two of the most prominent of these arguments were the fact that adults could serve in the military at the age of 18—a point that resonated strongly in the era of the Vietnam War—and that, if other states lowered their drinking ages, Michigan teenagers might just cross the border to procure alcohol, thereby raising the risk of traffic accidents. As described in the national case study, these concerns were similar to those which motivated the adoption of lower drinking ages in other states (Williams, 2011).

Factors Motivating the Increase

Unpacking the factors that led to the later increase in Michigan's minimum drinking age is more complicated, partly because of the complex nature of the policy changes themselves. The eventual increase to 21 was enacted through a public referendum; as the referendum movement grew stronger, the state legislature voted to increase the age to 19, but this did not blunt the movement's power and the referendum still passed (Legge, 1991).

In untangling the reasons for these increases, it is clear that, as already described, the decision to *lower* the drinking age, which came into force at the beginning of 1972, attracted controversy almost as soon as it was enacted, and such controversy only seemed to grow as time went on. In particular, interest groups helped raise public concern. The Michigan Parent Teacher Association, for example, began to push for an increase in the minimum age as early as the late 1970s (Begun, 1980). The drive for the referendum was spearheaded by the Michigan Council on Alcohol Problems, an alliance of parent-teacher associations, church groups, and other concerned organizations ("Group's aim ...", 1977). The group and its partner organizations gained more than 290,000 validated signatures on related petitions by September 1978, setting the stage for the national referendum (Kirley, 1978). Thus, as in the national case study, interest groups also played a fundamental role in encouraging legislative action in Michigan. This discovery offers further support for the idea that popular activism can affect alcohol policymaking, and echoes Weiss' (1983) ideas, discussed in Chapter 3, about the importance of competing interests in the policy process. The actions of the Michigan Council on Alcohol Problems also mirror those of the youth group in Sri Lanka which, as described in Chapter 5, secured 50,000 signatures to promote the passage of a 2006 bill that established a minimum legal drinking age of 21("New legislation in Sri Lanka", 2006). These similarities reveal that the power of such social movements in the alcohol policymaking process is not limited to a particular country, culture, or historical moment.

Of course, not all interest groups in Michigan supported the increase in the drinking age. Representatives of the alcohol industry in Michigan—in particular, alcohol retailers—were opposed to raising the legal drinking age and, through their lobbying, likely played a role in stalling efforts to raise the age to 21 in the state legislature (Toomey et al., 2009). In the run-up to the popular vote on the 1978 referendum, bar and food industry representatives opposed to the age increase formed the Michigan Committee for Age Responsibility, an organization that issued public warnings that an increase would bring economic and job losses (Legge, 1991).

The role of the alcohol industry in policymaking was discussed in detail in Chapter 3. Many stakeholders believe that the alcohol industry holds great sway over policy decisions in the US (Greenfield, Johnson, and Giesbrecht, 2004). If the alcohol industry did indeed help stall legislative efforts to raise the age to 21, then this case study offers support for the belief about the industry's significant power. However, the eventual passage of the referendum shows that the industry's influence is not infinite; in this case, it was outpaced by a popular vote.

In addition to the role of interest groups, a second similarity between Michigan's experiences and the national case study is the role that *research evidence* seems to have played in policymaking. In Michigan, one 1977 study showed that, after the state's minimum age was lowered to 18, alcohol-involved crashes rose among drivers aged 18 to 20 (Douglass and Freedman, 1977). The Michigan Council on Alcohol Problems' campaign to raise the age was motivated by broad worries over alcohol misuse among young people and not just traffic fatalities (Legge, 1991). To drive the campaign forward, research evidence was deployed and, in particular, the statistical claim that the policy could save 54 lives each year in the state—mainly due to reduced traffic deaths—was discussed in popular discourse (Toomey et al., 2009; Wagenaar, 1993), mirroring the later national debate in which, as described earlier, particularly salient statistics about the policy's potential consequences were often drawn upon.

As with the national case study, Michigan's example shows that evidence *can* play a role in alcohol policymaking. In that state, interest groups and popular movements promoted such evidence, as it supported the cause of raising the minimum age. In this example, therefore, the "two communities" of researchers and policymakers seem to have been brought together by interest groups and activists (Caplan, 1979; Rich, 1991, p. 324). The role of such groups and individuals in influencing the use of evidence in policymaking thus deserves greater attention from researchers.

Policy Consequences

As with the national policy, once the minimum age of 21 was enacted in Michigan it was quickly challenged in court. The Michigan Committee for Age Responsibility, the alcohol industry-led organization discussed earlier, joined with 18-to-20-year-olds to sue the state, arguing that the new law violated the Fourteenth Amendment's equal protection clause (Legge, 1991). The higher minimum age, however, was upheld in federal court, with the court citing scientific research indicating the law's potential effectiveness and rationality (Toomey et al., 2009). This development further illustrates the range of ways that research can influence the policy process; in addition to directly influencing legislators, it can also play a role in court decisions about policies.

A study by Filkins and Flora (1982) reveals that, after the minimum age of 21 was adopted in Michigan, alcohol-related traffic accidents among 18-to-20-year-olds decreased. A follow-up study conducted six years after the age increase, and based on a range of statistical measures, concluded that "the raised legal drinking age appears to have a long-term effect in reducing motor vehicle crash involvement among young drivers" (Wagenaar, 1986, p. 101). Although not as many studies have explored the effects of Michigan's minimum age law as have explored the effects of the national minimum age law, this evaluation offers some evidence of the Michigan policy's effectiveness.

Lingering Issues

The issue of the minimum drinking age in the US perennially attracts debate. Advocates of lowering the national minimum age continue to point out that individuals can serve in the military, vote, and marry before they are allowed to drink alcohol (Williams, 2011). One scholar has argued that although the minimum age of 21 does help reduce alcohol's social harms, "the claims of liberty have the upper hand over the claims of public health and safety" (Cook, 2010, p. 99). This statement illustrates that evidence is of course not the only factor that individuals must consider when taking policy positions; political, philosophical, and other beliefs can be more powerful than evidence, even for researchers.

In 2008 the Amethyst Initiative (2012), was founded, a movement that now has gained the support of at least 135 US college and university presidents, including the leaders of Dartmouth, Johns Hopkins, Middlebury, and the University of Maryland, College Park. The movement's goals include encouraging "informed and unimpeded debate on the 21-year-old drinking age" and its consequences (Amethyst Initiative, 2012). In response to the campaign, MADD reiterated its opposition to lowering the drinking age ("Amethyst Initiative, MADD ...", 2008), and encouraged members of the public to write to the college and university presidents and encourage them to withdraw their support from the Amethyst Initiative (Staudenmeier, 2011, p. 133). At the same time, the issue of enforcing the minimum drinking age has received greater attention from the federal government, with Congress in 2006 authorizing $18 million annually for efforts to reduce underage drinking (Hacker, 2006; "STOP Underage Drinking Act ...", 2006; p. 13).

Case Study: New Zealand

In 1999, New Zealand's government *reduced* the minimum age to purchase alcohol from 20 to 18, providing a fascinating case study that contrasts sharply with the American examples.[1] This section explores the history and motivations behind this policy change, examining whether the factors that influenced this change were

---

1   Strictly speaking, "New Zealand has no minimum legal drinking age" (Alcohol Advisory Council of New Zealand,n.d.); instead, the country maintains "a minimum legal purchase age" (Dalziel, 2005). Nevertheless, in common parlance, the term "minimum drinking age" is still sometimes used (e.g., Everitt and Jones, 2002; Fleming, 2006).

similar—or very different—from the factors that motivated the federal and state-level US policy changes described in the previous section.

History of the Policy Change

In 1996, an advisory committee was established to review the 1989 Sale of Liquor Act, which had adjusted alcohol licensing practices, and recommend potential policy changes to New Zealand's Ministry of Justice (Advisory Committee, 1997). The committee's 1997 report advanced a number of recommendations, including lowering the "minimum drinking age" to 18. According to the advisory committee (1997, Section 1.1) the potential change to the minimum drinking age was "the most controversial item" it had had to deal with, with 233 submissions about the issue from experts and the public. Of these 233 submissions, 112 advocated keeping the minimum age of 20.

Following the release of this report, a Sale of Liquor Amendment Bill was brought onto the legislative agenda and—after submissions from the public were reviewed by the Justice and Law Select Committee—MPs voted on different options. The successful options were then included in the final bill which was passed by Parliament in August 1999 (Hill, 2000). This bill became the 1999 Sale of Liquor Amendment Act and it came into force in December of that year, lowering the "minimum drinking age" to 18, with the exception that those under the age of 18 could be served alcohol in a licensed premises if they were given the alcohol by an accompanying parent or legal guardian (*Amendments to ...*, 1999). Lowering the minimum age was not the only change in alcohol policy ushered in by the new bill; other changes included allowing supermarkets to sell beer in addition to wine (Bellamy, 2003).

Factors Motivating the Policy Change

Exploring why the lower minimum age was adopted in New Zealand is particularly interesting, since, as Stockwell and Grunewald (2004, p. 221) have reported, the majority of the New Zealand public was against the change. Such opposition has persisted; indeed, a 2012 survey of New Zealanders found that a majority—54.4 percent of respondents—wanted the minimum age for purchasing alcohol to be raised to 20 in both restaurants and supermarkets, while just 19.4 percent thought the minimum age should remain at 18 for both restaurants/bars and supermarkets ("Drinking age should ...", 2012). This policy's adoption—and, at the time of writing, its persistence despite a lack of consistent and comprehensive public support, contrasts sharply with the discussion of public opinion and alcohol policy presented in Chapter 4, in which public opinion was said to play an important role in preventing the adoption of unpopular alcohol policies (Johnson et al., 2004). The New Zealand case study shows that a lack of public support does not always hinder the adoption of alcohol policies, even in a democratic context.

In addition to this lack of popular support, the policy was also distinguished by a dearth of endorsements from researchers and public health experts. Indeed, around the time of the bill's passage, many such researchers and experts argued that the age should not be lowered and that, instead, the current minimum age of 20 should be more strongly enforced (Kypri et al., 2006). As described above, just under half of the submissions from experts and the public to the advisory committee (1997) tasked with considering the age question advocated keeping the minimum age of 20. The majority of these submissions reasoned that increasing alcohol's availability would increase alcohol consumption, and subsequently increase alcohol misuse in society.

The submissions that advocated a *lower* age, however, typically argued that such a change would be easier to enforce (Advisory Committee, 1997). Although the official minimum age prior to 1999 was 20, as the Advisory Committee (1997, Section 1.1) noted, the law provided "many exceptions" to this minimum, and applied different regulations to areas of licensed premises that were deemed "supervised" or "restricted"—complicating efforts to enforce the measure. The need for clarity and more straightforward laws to ease enforcement can also be seen in a contemporaneous study (published in 1996) by scholars from the Alcohol and Public Research Unit at the University of Auckland; one key component of the study was a series of interviews conducted with officers involved in the alcohol licensing process in New Zealand communities (Hill and Stewart, 1996). According to the study's authors, these interviews revealed that "police efforts were undermined [by] lack of clarity and interpretation difficulties around ... exceptions to the legal drinking age of 20 when eating a meal or supervised by family members" (Hill and Stewart, 1996, p. 7). Although the interviewees expressed different opinions about what the minimum drinking age should be, "all interviewees wanted one clear legal drinking age, and the removal of exemptions and areas designated as age restricted or supervised, so that the Act could be easily understood and properly enforced by both licensees and police" (Hill and Stewart, 1996, pp. 7–8). It seems likely that this clear desire among many enforcement officers for straightforward, consistent, and more-easily-enforceable drinking age laws likely helped influence the policy's adoption. In a submission to the 1997 Advisory Committee, the New Zealand Police "did not make a recommendation as to a minimum drinking age, but did make a plea for the age selected to be made easier to enforce," according to the committee's report. Even seven years after the policy change, when the New Zealand Medical Association noted its opposition to raising the minimum age back to 20, the association's head suggested that better *enforcement* of the law would be more effective than any age change (Fleming, 2006). The practical issues of enforcement and implementation should therefore not be underestimated in any exploration of alcohol policies.

Additionally, other likely reasons for the adoption of the lower alcohol purchase age can be seen in comments made during a later (2005) parliamentary debate about a proposed bill that would raise the drinking age back to 20. In this debate, one politician observed that:

We have all heard the reasons being advanced as to why 18- and 19-year-olds should have the right to go into a pub and drink. They have the ability to marry. They have the legal ability to be in our armed forces and be sent overseas on peacekeeping missions or on missions to defend New Zealand ... At the very best, what [this bill] would achieve is to drive those 18-year-olds away from our hotels, to locations that are unpoliced and unsupervised. The important thing is that those 18- and 19-year-olds will drive their vehicles—their cars— to those particular locations, where they will still drink, and because they are unsupervised they will drink to excess, and then they will drive their cars home again. (Carter, 2005)

These arguments that 18-to-19-year olds already possessed many of the privileges and responsibilities of adulthood (in particular, they could serve in the military), and that a higher drinking age could *increase* the risk of alcohol-involved traffic accidents among young people, echo the arguments advanced in Michigan and many other US states during the Vietnam War Era, when these states lowered their drinking ages to 18 (Deloria and Wilkins, 1999; Legge, 1991; Williams, 2011). In 2012, New Zealand's Justice Minister said that she believed the minimum age should be kept at 18 for bars and restaurants, since "it's ridiculous if we have police officers aged 18 who go into bars enforcing the laws and they can't actually have a drink themselves in a bar" (as quoted in "Drinking age should ...", 2012). The emergence of these arguments in both the US in the 1960s and 1970s and in New Zealand in the 1990s and early twenty-first century shows that similar concerns can affect alcohol policies in very different cultural contexts.

Consequences of the Policy Change

As described previously, the 1999 Act did not merely lower the minimum age to purchase alcohol—it also enacted several other alcohol policy changes, such as allowing supermarkets to sell beer (Bellamy, 2003). This imposition of multiple policy changes at the same time complicates any effort to identify the consequences that *specifically* resulted from the reduction in the minimum age (as opposed to other policy changes or altered enforcement practices)—a difficulty that has been noted elsewhere (Lash, 2005). A second difficulty is that, according to a 2011 report published by the Office of the Prime Minister's Science Advisory Committee, "no clear plan was developed to evaluate the consequences" of lowering the minimum age and, unfortunately, this "lack of systematic evaluation of the evidence has complicated the process of policy debate and reform" (Fergusson and Boden, 2011, p. 242).

Despite these difficulties, it is clear that, following the 1999 legislation, the number of minors caught drinking in public or possessing alcohol rose (Marriott-Lloyd and Webb, 2002). Whether this rise indicates that consumption among young people increased, or that enforcement of alcohol laws increased, is a separate question, however. In support of the second explanation is the argument advanced by proponents of the lower minimum age that the policy would ease enforcement of the minimum age.

Some evidence suggests that some particular social harms among young people worsened after the policy change. Specifically, a study by Kypri and colleagues (2006) reveals that, in the period following the policy's enactment, alcohol-involved traffic accidents among 15-to-19-year olds were higher than they likely would have been if the law had not been changed. This increase reversed the longer-term fall in alcohol-involved traffic accidents among young drivers that had taken place earlier in the 1990s (Haines, 2005). Huckle, Pledger, and Casswell (2006) have concluded the lower minimum age may have increased rates of alcohol-impaired driving among 18-to-19-year-olds. In addition to traffic accidents, another useful data source is hospital statistics. A study of emergency department presentations at an urban New Zealand hospital suggests that the age reduction policy was associated with an increase in presentations by intoxicated 18- and 19-year-olds, as well as intoxicated 15-to-17-year olds (even though this latter group was not directly affected by the policy change) (Everitt and Jones, 2002).

This range of findings illustrates just how difficult it can be to evaluate— and, even more so, to predict—the consequences of a policy change. Indeed, the consequences of the 1999 Act, and the minimum age issue more generally, still prompt much debate in New Zealand. The issue's lingering controversy is illustrated by the 2006 proposal of a bill that would have reinstated a minimum purchase age of 20; although the bill was defeated on its second reading in Parliament, it prompted much heated discussion among politicians (Cagney and Palmer, 2007, p. 30).

Conclusion

Rarely do policy case studies offer as much comparative potential as the US and New Zealand examples discussed in this chapter. The examples show how societies facing many of the same societal pressures and problems can respond in opposite ways—with complex results. The examples also emphasize the complicated nature of policy decisions, and the range of reasons why research evidence might, and might not, influence policymaking.

One significant issue raised by both case studies is the role of popular opinion in alcohol-related policymaking. The Michigan case study highlights how popular movements can sometimes exert great influence in this area; in that state, a popular referendum overpowered the objections launched by the alcohol industry (Legge, 1991). Yet in New Zealand the lower drinking age was adopted even though a majority of the public seems to have been against the change (Stockwell and Grunewald, 2004, p. 221). This example illustrates that the link between public opinion and alcohol policy is not always straightforward; indeed, the influence of public opinion may depend upon the activities of vocal groups, such as the coalition of interest groups that gained prominence in Michigan.

A second issue that merits further discussion is that of *enforcement*. In order to be effective, an alcohol policy—such as a minimum drinking age—must be enforced. The issue of designing a policy that could be more easily enforced likely motivated the adoption of a lower drinking age in New Zealand. It is of course essential to consider the issue of enforcement when evaluating the outcomes of alcohol policies; indeed, a lack of enforcement can severely complicate policy evaluation efforts in this area. In the US, for example, Saltz and Fell (2012, p. 296) have observed that "enforcement of MLDA [the minimum legal drinking age] has been, at best, uneven"; this lack of consistent enforcement should be kept in mind when interpreting the outcomes of the US minimum age policy that were discussed earlier. Even more troublingly, data issued by the CDC (2006) suggests that many instances of alcohol-impaired driving—by all age groups—are never discovered by the police. Thus, the question of how to better *enforce* alcohol policies also applies to other alcohol policies beyond the minimum drinking age.

Thirdly, in addition to the deep differences between the US and New Zealand case studies, it is also important to note that significant cross-national differences in minimum drinking ages exist in other countries around the world. These differences have persisted despite international convergence in many other areas of alcohol policy. In Canada, a country with many similarities to the US and New Zealand, the minimum drinking age varies across the provinces, with an age of 18 in Manitoba, Alberta, and Quebec, and an age of 19 in the other provinces (Selvanathan and Selvanathan, 2005, p. 296). At the time of writing, in the UK, the minimum age is 18, although 16- and 17-year-olds can drink wine and beer (but not spirits) in a pub if they are eating a meal, and the alcohol is purchased by an accompanying adult ("Children and drink ...", 2007). The British Medical Association does not officially endorse raising the legal drinking age to 21, but a spokesperson for the organization has noted that "evidence from America clearly demonstrates that raising the legal drinking age has a significant positive effect on alcohol-related problems" (as quoted in de Castella, 2012). The British Medical Association's position underlines how evidence and policies from one country can inform the debate about this issue in other countries.

The wider issue of cross-national policy diffusion, and the work of Dobbin, Simmons, and Garrett (2007), as well as other scholars in this area, was explored in detail in Chapter 3. Dobbin and colleagues have explored how countries can learn from other countries' policy experiences; if one country adopts a policy that seems to be successful, other countries will want to bring that policy to their own territory. Conversely, if one country adopts a policy that seems to be a failure, other countries will know to steer clear of that approach. This same process of learning and cross-national influence can be detected in an interesting political speech that directly relates to both case studies discussed in this chapter. In 2007, a Texas Congressman delivered a speech in the US House of Representatives in which he argued that the American minimum drinking age should not be lowered; specifically, the Congressman asserted that:

> In 1999, New Zealand lowered its drinking age from 20 to 18. Not only did the alcohol-involved crash rate increase among 18- and 19-year-olds, but also among 15- to 17-year-olds. It is absurd to think that this would not happen in the United States were we to take the easy path. (Poe, 2007, p. 16752)

This example not only highlights a further intersection between the two case studies discussed in this chapter, but also illustrates how countries' experiences with alcohol policies can resonate far beyond their borders.

Chapter 8
Concluding Thoughts

The social harms of alcohol misuse are immense, and societies throughout history and around the world have grappled with the question of how to best combat them. Although an ever-growing body of research has explored which policies are most effective, the question of how to best facilitate the adoption and implementation of such policies deserves more attention from researchers. Research evidence is just one of the many factors that can influence alcohol policies; political, economic, cultural, historical, and other forces frequently play important roles. This book's primary aim has been to explore diverse examples of the alcohol policymaking process in greater detail to better identify these various factors. The use of case studies from different time periods and world regions illustrates that some findings about alcohol policymaking are widely applicable, while others are critically dependent upon specific historical or cultural contexts. Not all of the book's findings can be reviewed in this chapter; however, a number of particularly salient discoveries deserve restatement and further examination.

Globalization is Driving Significant Changes in Alcohol Policy

One of the most prominent, recurrent findings in this book has been the impact of globalizing forces on alcohol policy. This book's introduction discussed the WHO's international approach to tackling alcohol's social harms—in particular, its 2010 Global Strategy, which encourages the international adoption of price incentives for non-alcoholic drinks, minimum age limits for the purchase of alcohol, and other policies (pp. 8–23). The WHO's international-focused efforts in this area have been longstanding; indeed, the organization's interest in the international dissemination of evidence-based strategies to combat alcohol's social harms dates back several decades (Jernigan et al., 2000; WHO, 2007).

In addition to the WHO, other supranational bodies, such as the EU, have also contributed to cross-national harmonization in alcohol policies. The case study of Sweden illustrates the power of such influence, and offers support for Dobbin and colleagues' (2007) idea, outlined in Chapter 3, that international organizations can be important drivers of policy diffusion. Although not an example of supranational pressures, the case study of the US minimum drinking age similarly reveals how larger governmental decisions can sharply affect regional communities' efforts to regulate alcohol.

This discussion prompts the more general question of whether it is possible for regions or communities to maintain distinct alcohol policies in an interlinked world. This question was exemplified most visibly in this book's introduction, through the case study of the Pine Ridge Reservation in South Dakota. Although alcohol is prohibited on the Reservation's grounds, its rampant availability in a nearby town has undermined this ban, and alcohol-related social harms are now rife at Pine Ridge (Williams, 2012). The Pine Ridge case study thus underlines the difficulties communities can face when attempting to maintain distinct alcohol policies within a connected world—a task that will likely become increasingly difficult as globalizing forces strengthen.

Cultural Differences Matter, Although Policies Don't Always Account for Them

Related to the discussion of globalization is another key theme: cultural differences. Although such differences can sharply affect attitudes to alcohol and drinking patterns, alcohol policies—particularly when implemented through a globalized framework—cannot always take them into account. Yet such differences must be considered when exploring questions of how to most effectively migrate policies from one region or country to another. As discussed in Chapter 3, Dolowitz and Marsh (2000) have examined the problems that hinder or prevent the successful diffusion of policies across societies or countries. According to Dolowitz and Marsh, one such problem involves policymakers and other stakeholders overlooking the fact that a policy was designed to fit a different political or economic system, or was designed to achieve specific goals, which do not apply in the new society or country. The importance of local context can be seen in the Sri Lankan case study, discussed in Chapter 5. In that country, Protestant missionaries encouraged temperance in the late nineteenth century, yet temperance ideas did not achieve real influence until they were promoted within a Buddhist framework by native Sri Lankans (Rogers, 1989), a finding which highlights the importance of adapting policies to suit local contexts. In the specific realm of alcohol policy, the need to tailor policies to fit the unique needs and characteristics of a particular society has gained increasing recognition in some countries (e.g., Samarasinghe, 2006, p. 628). Societies have unique needs, and even the cost-effectiveness of various policy options can depend on the specific range of problems experienced by a particular society (Chisholm et al., 2004).

More broadly, the power of alcohol-related cultural traditions to shape reactions to alcohol policies can be seen in the deeply disapproving (but partially tongue-in-cheek) reaction by some British commentators to nudge theorist Richard Thaler's suggestion that Britons should eschew the practice of buying rounds of alcohol (e.g., Pelling, 2011). The negative reactions of such commentators illustrate just how difficult it can be to challenge ingrained cultural traditions and the tide of history. History's influence can also be detected in the fact that historical alcohol events and policies, such as the eighteenth-century British gin craze and Prohibition in the early twentieth-century US, are still referenced in contemporary discussions about alcohol (e.g., Humphrys, 2010; Newman, 2012). These references underline the significant role that cultural memory—specifically, societal interpretations of past phenomena—can play in shaping reactions to alcohol policy.

Public Opinion is Often, But Not Always, Significant

Culture and public opinion are often closely intertwined, and the case studies presented in this book illustrate how public opinion can play a crucial, but often complex, role in the alcohol policymaking process. Chapter 4 introduced important previous studies about public opinion and alcohol policies, including Johnson and colleagues' (2004, pp. 747–8) description about how proposals to increase national excise taxes on alcohol in the US in the 1990s were not adopted in part because of the lack of public support. The power of public opinion can also be seen in the Soviet Union case study, discussed in Chapter 5, where the prohibition policy instituted by Gorbachev became increasingly unpopular, and was undermined by the illegal production of alcohol (Kondakov, 1988; Nemtsov, 2011; "Prohibition, Soviet style", 1990). The case study of the minimum age policy in Michigan also shows how popular movements, propelled by influential groups, can affect alcohol policymaking; in that case, a popular referendum on the minimum age policy overpowered the objections launched by the alcohol industry (Legge, 1991).

Yet public opinion's role is not always as straightforward, as the case study of lowering the minimum drinking age in New Zealand illustrates. This policy was adopted even though a majority of the public seems to have been against the change (Stockwell and Grunewald, 2004, p. 221). In Chapter 7, numerous alternative factors were examined that may have encouraged the adoption of the lower minimum age, and their triumph illustrates that public opinion's influence is not always *dominant* in the alcohol policy process—a key lesson of this book's analysis.

Public opinion's role in alcohol policymaking is further complicated by the fact that it is subject to cultural forces. Public opinions and perceptions of alcohol-related social harms differ widely among societies; for example, Jayne, Valentine, and Holloway (2010) found that, in a rural region of the UK, harmful drinking was seen by some residents as an urban problem, a finding that MacLean (2011, p. 689) has contrasted with the situation in Australia, "where alcohol consumption is generally higher in rural and regional than in urban areas."

Perhaps not surprisingly, public opinion is also often more supportive of less intrusive (but also often less effective) policies to combat alcohol's social harms, such as alcohol education. In contrast, public opinion is typically less supportive of more invasive strategies such as raising alcohol taxes or restricting the number of alcohol outlets, even though they might be more effective and evidence-based (Giesbrecht et al., 2007). Thus, when examining the role of evidence in alcohol policymaking, it is essential to also explore whether policies supported by evidence are also supported by public opinion. The additional question of whether public opinion could be effectively mobilized to facilitate the adoption of evidence-based alcohol policies deserves greater attention from researchers.

Interest Groups and Policy Entrepreneurs Can Play Key Roles

In addition to public opinion, the case studies presented in this book also offer insight into the ways in which interest groups and "policy entrepreneurs"—individuals with particular "connections" and "persistence" that allow them to bring policies onto the legislative agenda (Kingdon, 2003, pp. 180–82)—can influence alcohol policymaking.

The first of these themes—the importance of interest groups—is clearly illustrated in the case study of the national adoption of the minimum drinking age in the US, explored in Chapter 7. In that case study, a victim-oriented advocacy group, MADD, played a key role (Treuthart, 2005, pp. 108–9; Voas and Fell, 2010). Similarly, many decades earlier, organized temperance groups helped facilitate the adoption of Prohibition in the early-twentieth-century US (Schrad, 2010). These kinds of socially- and ideologically-driven groups are of course not the only interest groups that can significantly affect alcohol policymaking. Economic interest groups can also exert influence, as shown by Bakke and Endal's (2010) findings, discussed in Chapter 3, about the alcohol industry in four sub-Saharan African countries. Miller and colleagues (2011) have similarly explored the role of Australia's alcohol industry in promoting strategies that would not harm the industry's profits. In many countries, the alcohol industry is an important contributor to the national economy. To offer just one example of this, the brewing and pub industry is worth £28 billion a year to the British economy, and supports more than half-a-million jobs (Brown, 2012). All of these substantive findings offer support for Weiss' (1983) idea—outlined in Chapter 3—that competing interests shape policymaking. Ritter and Bammer (2010) have previously applied Weiss' ideas to alcohol policymaking, and many of the case studies presented in this book similarly highlight the relevance of her insights.

In addition to interest groups, the second theme that deserves discussion here is that of policy entrepreneurs, perhaps most clearly illustrated in the discussion of the history of Swedish alcohol policies advanced in Chapter 6. That historical discussion highlighted the role of Ivan Bratt, a Stockholm doctor, who responded to rising public concerns about alcohol by proposing several far-reaching and influential policies targeting alcohol's social harms (Eriksen, 2003; Schrad, 2010; Shanks and Tilley, 1987, pp. 193–4). Similarly, as described in Chapter 5, in Sri Lanka, although the 1904 movement was not successful in instituting its ultimate goal of prohibition, the movement did highlight the power of policy entrepreneurs—in this case, a number of individuals from the Sri Lankan elite who had few other opportunities to exert true political leadership under colonial rule (Rogers, 1989). These elites helped bring greater attention to the societal problem of alcohol misuse, and increased the national salience of the prohibition question.

The fact that both interest groups *and* policy entrepreneurs featured in this book's case studies is important as it shows that key ideas from general policymaking theories—namely, Weiss and Kingdon's theories—are also relevant in the specific area of alcohol policymaking.

Research Evidence is Just One Source of Influence

Although—as Ritter and Bammer (2010, p. 353) have observed—a rational model of policymaking would naturally specify a key role for research evidence in the policy process, Weiss (1983) has cautioned that research evidence is not the only kind of "evidence" that policymakers often consider. Other kinds of "evidence" that are routinely deployed to influence policymaking include anecdotes, appeals to common sense, rival claims, and other kinds of arguments advanced by stakeholders in the policymaking process. As Choi and colleagues (2005, p. 633) have argued, policymakers sometimes only "look for evidence to support their claims." Johnson and colleagues' (2004) study of alcohol policymaking in the US offers support for this argument. In that study's interviews, some policy stakeholders admitted to using research for rhetorical purposes such as supporting their established policy positions or increasing their public popularity, rather than for informative purposes (pp. 744–5).

The questions of what counts as evidence, and whether there are some kinds of evidence that should *not* influence policy, were explored in detail in Chapter 3. However, taken as a whole, the case studies presented in the book reveal that policymakers rarely have the time or ability to critically review the results of rigorous, long-term evaluations of policies or programs; indeed, for many policies, such evaluations don't even exist. The case study of the national minimum drinking age, discussed in Chapter 7, highlights many of the practical complexities of evidence's role in alcohol policymaking. Although the case study might initially be seen as an encouraging example of evidence-based policymaking, since research appeared to influence policy action (Toomey and Rosenfeld, 1996; Voas and Fell, 2010, p. 18), the quality and comprehensiveness of some of the studies relied upon during this period has been questioned (Males, 1986, pp. 181–2; Treuthart, 2005, p. 110). Thus, even when evidence *does* influence policymaking, questions about that evidence's rigor—and whether it *should* have influenced policy—can sometimes remain.

Finally, although this book has emphasized the importance of evidence-based policymaking, it should be recognized that evidence cannot—and should not be— the only driver of policy. Sometimes other considerations trump evidence; for example, as discussed in the previous chapter, at least one scholar has admitted that although he believes a minimum drinking age of 21 does help reduce alcohol's social harms, he feels that "the claims of liberty have the upper hand over the claims of public health and safety" (Cook, 2010, p. 99). This quotation is worth repeating here since it serves as a reminder not to forget the very real other pressures and values—in addition to evidence of effectiveness—that shape policymakers' decisions.

Underground Drinking Deserves Greater Attention

Many of the policies examined in this book aim to reduce alcohol's social harms by controlling or limiting access to alcohol. Before concluding, it is essential to consider one concern that has often been raised about such policies—that they might simply encourage illegal and dangerous "underground" alcohol consumption. Such concerns are evident in the Soviet Union case study discussed in Chapter 5, where the crackdown on legal alcohol increased demand for homemade alcohol. Tragically, according to one estimate, in 1988 alone some 11,000 people died as a result of drinking such underground alcohol ("Prohibition, Soviet style", 1990). This increase in underground drinking "brought a heavy strain on the police, the judiciary and the penal institutions", placing further strains on Soviet society (Partanen, 1993, p. 130S). The underground criminal enterprises and violence that flourished after the establishment of American Prohibition in the early twentieth century are legendary. Similarly, but less dramatically, in Australia, Hall and Hunter (1995, p. 9) have argued that the strict laws governing the trading hours of alcohol outlets—laws that were in place for much of the first half of the twentieth century—encouraged the development of underground, illegal drinking, known as "sly grogging."

It is, unsurprisingly, extremely difficult to estimate the prevalence of illegal alcohol production and consumption. However, in some areas at particular historical moments, this activity might be very high indeed. For example, a poll conducted in Sweden in the 1970s, found that just over a fifth of Swedes had tried illegal alcohol (Doos, 1982).

Despite the inherent difficulties of measuring underground alcohol consumption, given the potential health risks posed, persistence in forecasting and measuring the risk of such activity is important. More broadly, however, this discussion serves as a reminder that alcohol policies, such as American Prohibition or Gorbachev's anti-alcohol campaign in the Soviet Union, can have *unintended* and sometimes fatal consequences. When evaluating alcohol policies it is thus essential to not only consider whether such policies achieve their intended goals, but also whether *unintended* (and potentially harmful) outcomes also result from their enactment.

A Final Case Study: Diadema, Brazil

Although this book has highlighted many of alcohol policymaking's challenges, and some perceived failures, it should be remembered that effective policies can reap massive social benefits. This book's final case study shows that "success stories" are indeed possible.

In 1999, Diadema was a poverty-stricken city in the state of São Paulo with one of the highest murder rates in Brazil—103 homicides annually per 100,000 residents, a rate more than 11 times higher than that of New York City in the same year (Duailibi et al., 2007, p. 2276; US Department of Justice, 2000). A new mayor took office in Diadema in 2001 and, frustrated with the continual violence, directed researchers to map the locations of crimes and note the times when they occurred (Downie, 2006a). The map revealed that 60 percent of murders took place between 11pm and 6am, typically in areas with multiple bars and nightclubs; many of these murders were spontaneous rather than premeditated (Pacific Institute for Research and Evaluation, 2004, pp. 5–6). The city government responded swiftly to the findings. In July 2002, a new policy was introduced which forbade the city's bars, restaurants, nightclubs, and other establishments from serving alcohol after 11pm (Anderson, Chisholm, and Fuhr, 2009, p. 2239). A rigorous administrative enforcement regime and substantial publicity helped increase awareness of the policy among residents and Diadema's more than 4,000 alcohol-serving establishments (Downie, 2006a; Gorgulho and Da Ros, 2006). Specifically, brochures were circulated to Diadema's households and radio announcements were made, and some 98 percent of the local population claimed to be aware of the new restriction; additionally, three months before the law was adopted, alcohol retailers were called upon to sign a document indicating they understood the law's content (Pacific Institute for Research and Evaluation, 2004, p. 6; "Reducing homicide ...", n.d.). Additionally, to reduce the risk of corruption, in the enforcement units that patrolled the city after 11pm looking for violators, only the team leader was aware of the planned itinerary, and inspectors and police always travelled together (Downie, 2006b). Following the discussion of public opinion earlier in this chapter, it is also important to note that, just before the policy was adopted, over 80 percent of the local community was found to support it—a fact that likely facilitated the policy's introduction and effective enforcement ("Reducing homicide ...", n.d).

In the first three years after the policy's enactment, homicide rates fell by an astonishing 44 percent (Duailibi et al., 2007, p. 2277). According to research by the Pacific Institute for Research and Evaluation (2004, p. 4): "Diadema is preventing eleven murders each month as a direct result of its adoption and enforcement of the new alcohol policy." This increased level of safety encouraged companies to operate in the area and for 20 continuous months, Diadema had the highest number of jobs created in the state of São Paulo (Downie, 2006a). This development illustrates that economic growth can be a potential byproduct of alcohol policies.

Of course, Diadema's restrictive sales policy cannot take sole credit for all of the social benefits the locality experienced during this period. Indeed, during this period a number of other policy and societal changes also took place, which may have also contributed to the overall decreases (Manso, Faria, and Gall, 2005). Nevertheless, Diadema's example shows that efforts to reduce alcohol-related social harms *can* succeed. The example also illustrates that alcohol-related social harms are often intertwined within a constellation of other social harms which must also often be addressed by other community interventions.

Unsurprisingly, Diadema's "success story" has received significant positive attention around the world; a Google search of the terms "Diadema," "Brazil," and "alcohol," returns more than a million hits. The case study has also attracted attention from the Pan American Health Organization (a regional office of the WHO) (Monteiro, 2007, p. 25) and the prominent US newsmagazine *Time* (Downie, 2006b), among other international organizations and news sources.

Many scholars have dreamed of creating Diademas all over the world: places where effective alcohol policies, based upon rigorous evidence, are employed to successfully reduce alcohol's social harms. Despite such dreams, relatively scant research has examined *how* such policies can be developed, adopted, and implemented, and for every Diadema many less successful examples can be found. Only by examining the factors that have been found to facilitate, and hinder, the use of research evidence in alcohol policymaking, can scholars, policy proponents, politicians, and other policy actors encourage the adoption and implementation of effective, evidence-based alcohol strategies.

Bibliography[1]

A Soviet alcohol problem? U.S. has one just as big. (1990, 22 October). *San Diego Union-Tribune*, p. B7. Retrieved from www.newsbank.com.

Aaron, P., and Musto, D. (1981). Temperance and prohibition in America: A historical overview. In M.H. Moore and D.R. Gerstein (eds), *Alcohol and Public Policy: Beyond The Shadow of Prohibition* (pp. 127–81). Washington, DC: National Academies Press.

Abel, E. (1997). Was the fetal alcohol syndrome recognized in the ancient Near East? *Alcohol and Alcoholism, 32*(1), 3–7.

Abel, E. (2001). The gin epidemic: Much ado about what? *Alcohol and Alcoholism, 36*(5), 401–5.

Abel, E.L. (2006). Fetal alcohol syndrome: A cautionary note. *Current Pharmaceutical Design, 12*, 1521–9.

Academy of Medical Sciences, The (2004). *Calling Time: The Nation's Drinking as a Major Health Issue*. London: Author.

Adrian, M., Ferguson, B.S., and Her, M. (2001). Can alcohol price policies be used to reduce drunk driving? Evidence from Canada. *Substance Use and Misuse, 36*(13), 1923–57.

Advisory Committee (1997). *Liquor Review Report of the Advisory Committee*. Wellington, New Zealand: Ministry of Justice. Retrieved from http://www.justice.govt.nz/publications/publications-archived/1997/liquor-review-report-of-the-advisory-committee-march-1997.

Ahlström, S., Karlsson, T., and Österberg, E. (2004). Alcohol policy on the agenda of the European Union. In R. Müller and H. Klingemann (eds), *From Science to Action? 100 Years Later—Alcohol Policies Revisited* (pp. 5–14). Dordrecht, the Netherlands: Kluwer Academic Publishers.

Akyeampong, E.K. (1996). *Drink, Power, and Cultural Change: A Social History of Alcohol in Ghana, c. 1800 to Recent Times*. Portsmouth, NH: Heinemann.

Alavaikko, M., and Österberg, E. (2000). The influence of economic interests on alcohol control policy: A case study from Finland. *Addiction, 95*(s4), s565–s579.

Albala, K. (2006). To your health: Wine as food and medicine in mid-sixteenth-century Italy. In M.P. Holt (ed.), *Alcohol: A Social and Cultural History* (pp. 11–24). Oxford, UK: Berg.

Alcohol (2009). In D. Hayes and R. Laudan (eds), *Food and Nutrition* (vol. 1) (pp. 33–6). Tarrytown, NY: Marshall Cavendish.

---

1 All web addresses listed in the bibliography were accessible as of February 2013.

Alcohol Advisory Council of New Zealand (n.d.). The drinking age laws. Retrieved from http://www.alac.org.nz/legislation-policy/sale-liquor-act/ drinking-age-laws.

Alcohol Policy Network in Europe (2012). Welcome to APN. Retrieved from http://www.alcoholpolicynetwork.eu/home/welcom-to-apn.

Alcohol warnings effectiveness discussed (2012, 22 May). *Sky News (Australian News Channel Pty Ltd)*. Retrieved from http://www.skynews.com.au/health/article.aspx?id=752804&vId=.

Allen, M.D., Pettus, C., and Haider-Markel, D.P. (2004). Making the national local: Specifying the conditions for national government influence on state policymaking. *State Politics and Policy Quarterly*, *4*(3), 318–44.

Amaro, H., Dai, J. Arévalo, S., et al. (2007). Effects of integrated trauma treatment on outcomes in a racially/ethnically diverse sample of women in urban community-based substance abuse treatment. *Journal of Urban Health*, *84*(4), 508–22.

Ambler, C.H. (2003). Southern Africa. In J.S. Blocker, D.M. Fahey, and I.R. Tyrrell (eds), *Alcohol and Temperance in Modern History: A Global Encyclopedia* (pp. 10–13). Santa Barbara, CA: ABC-CLIO.

Amendments to the 1989 Sale of Liquor Act. (1999). Ministry of Justice: Wellington, New Zealand. Retrieved from http://www.justice.govt.nz/ publications/publications-archived/1999/amendments-to-the-1989-sale-of-liquor-act/publication.

American Psychiatric Association (1980). *Diagnostic and Statistical Manual of Mental Disorders* (3rd ed.). Washington, DC: Author.

American Psychiatric Association (1994). *Diagnostic and Statistical Manual of Mental Disorders* (4th ed.). Washington, DC: Author.

American Psychiatric Association. (2000). *Diagnostic and Statistical Manual of Mental Disorders* (4th ed., text rev.). Washington, DC: Author.

Amethyst initiative (2012). About. Retrieved from http://www. theamethystinitiative.org.

Amethyst initiative, MADD disagree over drinking age. (2008, 30 September). *The August Chronicle*. Retrieved from www.chronicle.augusta.com.

AMPHORA (2010). The AMPHORA project. Retrieved from http://www. amphoraproject.net.

Anderson, P. (2008). *Reducing Drinking and Driving in Europe*. Hamm, Germany: German Centre for Addiction Issues.

Anderson, P., Chisholm, D., and Fuhr, D.C. (2009). Effectiveness and cost-effectiveness of policies and programmes to reduce the harm caused by alcohol. *The Lancet*, *373*(9682), 2234–46.

Anderson, S.C., and Hibbs, V.K. (1992). Alcoholism in the Soviet Union. *International Social Work*, *35*, 441–53.

Andréasson. S., Nilsson, R., and Bränström, R. (2009). Monitoring alcohol and alcohol related problems in Sweden. *Contemporary Drug Problems*, *36*, 625–42.

Ariyoshi, H. (2010). An evaluation of alcohol dependence prevention measures at a Japanese newspaper company. *American Association of Occupational Health Nurses Journal, 58*(10), 433–6.

Armstrong, E.M., and Abel, E.L. (2000). Fetal alcohol syndrome: The origins of a moral panic. *Alcohol and Alcoholism, 35*(3), 276–82.

Arriola, K.R. J., Usdan, S., Mays, D., et al. (2009). Reliability and validity of the Alcohol Consequences Expectations Scale. *American Journal of Health Behavior, 33*(5), 504–12.

Arthurson, R. (1985). Evaluation of random breath testing. Research Note RN 10/85. Sydney, Australia: Traffic Authority of New South Wales.

Associated Press (1990, 15 October). Soviets battle alcohol problem. *The Windsor Star*, p. D7. Retrieved from www.proquest.com.

Associated Press (2011, 5 January). British pub glass size rules relaxed to allow Australian-size schooners. *The Australian*. Retrieved from http://www. theaustralian.com.au/news/world/british-pub-glass-size-rules-relaxed-to-allow-australian-size-schooners/story-e6frg6so-1225982261326.

Astley, S.J. (2004). Fetal alcohol syndrome prevention in Washington State: Evidence of success. *Paediatric and Perinatal Epidemiology, 18*, 344–51.

Aylward, C. (2012, 9 May). Cracking down on young drunk drivers. *The Telegram*. Retrieved from http://www.thetelegram.com/News/Local/2012-05-09/article-2974371/Cracking-down-on-young-drunk-drivers/1.

Babor, T.F. (2002). Linking science to policy: The role of international collaborative research. *Alcohol Research and Health, 26*(1), 66–74.

Babor, T.F. (2004). Alcohol policy and the public good: As simple as one, two, three? In R. Müller and H. Klingemann (eds), *From Science to Action? 100 Years Later—Alcohol Policies Revisited* (pp. 29–48). Dordrecht, the Netherlands: Kluwer Academic Publishers.

Babor, T.F., and Caetano, R. (2005). Evidence-based alcohol policy in the Americas: Strengths, weaknesses, and future challenges. *Revista Panamericana de Salud Pública, 18*(4/5), 327–37.

Babor, T.F., Caetano, R., Casswell, S., et al. (2003). *Alcohol: No Ordinary Commodity: Research and Public Policy*. Oxford, UK: Oxford University Press.

Baer, J.S., Sampson, P.D., Barr, H.M., et al. (2003). A 21-year longitudinal analysis of the effects of prenatal alcohol exposure on young adult drinking. *Archives of General Psychiatry, 60*, 377–85.

Bagnardi, V., Blangiardo, M., La Vecchia, C., and Corrao, G. (2001). Alcohol consumption and the risk of cancer: A meta-analysis. *Alcohol Research and Health, 25*(4), 263–70.

Bakke, Ø., and Endal, D. (2010). Alcohol policies out of context: Drinks industry supplanting government role in alcohol policies in sub-Saharan Africa. *Addiction, 105*, 22–8.

Baltagi, B.H., and Geishecker, I. (2006). Rational alcohol addiction: Evidence from the Russian longitudinal monitoring survey. *Health Economics, 15*, 893–914.

Banerjee, A., and Duflo, E. (2011). *Poor Economics: A Radical Rethinking of the Way to Fight Global Poverty*. New York: PublicAffairs.

Bärnighausen, T., and Bloom, D.E. (2011). The global health workforce. In S. Glied and P.C. Smith (eds), *The Oxford Handbook of Health Economics* (pp. 486–519). Oxford, UK: Oxford University Press.

Barrow, M. (2003). Band of hope. In J.S. Blocker, D.M. Fahey, and I.R. Tyrrell (eds), *Alcohol and Temperance in Modern History: A Global Encyclopedia* (pp. 86–7). Santa Barbara, CA: ABC-CLIO.

Barry, J., and Armstrong, R. (2011). *Towards A Framework For Implementing Evidence Based Alcohol interventions: A Health Service Executive Report*. Dublin, Ireland: Health Service Executive. Retrieved from http://www.hse.ie/eng/services/Publications/topics/alcohol/towards%20a%20Framework%20for%20Implementing%20Evidence%20Based%20Alcohol%20interventions.pdf.

Beauvais, F. (1992). The need for community consensus as a condition of policy implementation in the reduction of alcohol abuse on Indian reservations. *American Indian and Alaska Native Mental Health Research*, 4(3), 77–81.

Beccaria, F., and White, H.R. (2012). Underage drinking in Europe and North America. In P. De Witte and M.C. Mitchell (eds), *Underage Drinking: A Report On Drinking in the Second Decade of Life in Europe and North America* (pp. 21–78). Louvain-la-Neuve, Belgium: Presses Universitaires de Louvain.

Beck, U. (1992). *Risk Society: Towards a New Modernity*. London: SAGE.

Beckett, K. (1995). Fetal rights and "crack moms": Pregnant women in the war on drugs. *Contemporary Drug Problems*, 22, 587–612.

Begun, A.L. (1980). Social policy evaluation: An example from drinking age legislation. *Evaluation and Program Planning*, 3, 165–70.

Beirness, D.J. (2001). Alcohol involvement in snowmobile operator fatalities in Canada. *Canadian Journal of Public Health*, 92(5), 359–60.

Bell, H.M. (1938). *Youth Tell Their Story*. Washington, DC: American Council on Education.

Bellamy, P. (2003). *Alcohol and New Zealand Teenagers*. Wellington, New Zealand: Parliamentary Library. Retrieved from http://www.parliament.nz/NR/rdonlyres/F1C84C49-7A9E-4F65-90DF-BEBDFCAE9BFD/488/0311Alcohol92.pdf.

Bengtsson, H. (1938). The temperance movement and temperance legislation in Sweden. *Annals of the American Academy of Political and Social Science*, 197, 134–53.

Bennett, T., and Holloway, K. (2010). Is UK drug policy evidence based? *International Journal of Drug Policy*, 21, 411–17.

Bentzen, J., and Smith, V. (2004). The Nordic countries. In K. Anderson (ed.), *The World's Wine Markets: Globalization at Work* (pp. 141–60). Cheltenham, UK: Edward Elgar.

Bergen, G., Shults, R.A., and Rudd, R.A. (2011). Vital signs: Alcohol-impaired driving among adults—United States, 2010. *Journal of the American Medical Association: Morbidity and Mortality Weekly Report*, 306(20), 1351–6.

Berger, K., Ajani, U.A., Kase, C.S., et al. (1999). Light-to-moderate alcohol consumption and the risk of stroke among US male physicians. *New England Journal of Medicine, 341*(21): 1557–64.

Berkwitz, S.C. (2006). Buddhism in Sri Lanka: Practice, protest, and preservation. In S.C. Berkwitz (ed.), *Buddhism in World Cultures: Comparative Perspectives* (pp. 45–72). Santa Barbara, CA: ABC-CLIO.

Berridge, V., Herring, R., and Thom, B. (2009). Binge drinking: A confused concept and its contemporary history. *Social History of Medicine, 22*(3), 597–607.

Berry, F.S. (1994). Sizing up state policy innovation research. *Policy Studies Journal, 22*, 442–56.

Bevanger, L. (2005, 22 November). Swedish ads urge EU alcohol curbs. *BBC News*. Retrieved from http://news.bbc.co.uk/1/hi/world/africa/4458622.stm.

Bilefsky, D. (2007, 6 June). EU court loosens grip of Sweden on alcohol: State-owned monopoly loses its control. *International Herald Tribune*, p. 13. Retrieved from www.proquest.com.

Birckmayer, J., and Hemenway, D. (1999). Minimum-age drinking laws and youth suicide, 1970–1990. *American Journal of Public Health, 89*, 1365–8.

Bjerre, B. (2003). An evaluation of the Swedish ignition interlock program. *Traffic Injury Prevention, 4*, 98–104.

Blainey, A. (2003). Australia. In J.S. Blocker, D.M. Fahey, and I.R. Tyrrell (eds), *Alcohol and Temperance in Modern History: A Global Encyclopedia* (pp. 75–9). Santa Barbara, CA: ABC-CLIO.

Bond, G.D. (1988). *The Buddhist Revival in Sri Lanka*. Columbia, SC: University of South Carolina Press.

Bondi, M.W., Drake, A.I., and Grant, I. (1998). Verbal learning and memory in alcohol abusers and polysubstance abusers with concurrent alcohol abuse. *Journal of the International Neuropsychological Society, 4*(4), 319–28.

Bongers, I.M.B. (1998). *Problem Drinking Among the General Population: A Public Health Issue*. Rotterdam, the Netherlands: Instituut voor Verslavingsonderzoek.

Borsay, P. (2007, September). Binge drinking and moral panics: Historical parallels? *History and Policy*. Retrieved from http://www.historyandpolicy. org/papers/policy-paper-62.html.

Botolo, T. (2012, 9 May). Traffic deaths, crime up by 44 percent—Malawi police. *Nyasa Times*. Retrieved from http://www.nyasatimes.com/malawi/ 2012/05/09/traffic-deaths-crime-up-by-44-percent-malawi-police.

Brady, M. (2000). Alcohol policy issues for indigenous people in the United States, Canada, Australia and New Zealand. *Contemporary Drug Problems, 27*, 435–509.

Brand, D.A., Saisana, M., Rynn, L.A., et al. (2007). Comparative analysis of alcohol control policies in 30 countries. *PLoS Medicine, 4*, e151.

Brazil Senate approves controversial World Cup law. (2012, 10 May). *BBC News*. Retrieved from http://www.bbc.co.uk/news/world-latin-america-18017540.

British Heart Foundation (2012). Alcohol and heart disease. Retrieved from http://www.bhf.org.uk/heart-health/prevention/healthy-eating/alcohol.aspx.

British Medical Association (2011). *Social Determinants of Health: What Doctors Can Do*. London: Author. Retrieved from http://www.bma.org.uk/images/socialdeterminantshealth_tcm41-209805.pdf.

British Medical Association (BMA) Board of Science (2008). *Alcohol Misuse: Tackling the UK Epidemic*. London: Author.

British Museum, The (n.d.). Highlights: William Hogarth, *Beer Street* and *Gin Lane*, two prints. Retrieved from http://www.britishmuseum.org/explore/highlights/highlight_objects/pd/w/william_hogarth,_beer_street.aspx.

Bromley, R.D.F., and Nelson, A.L. (2002). Alcohol-related crime and disorder across urban space and time: Evidence from a British city. *Geoforum, 33*, 239–54.

Brown, P. (2012, 23 March). Britain's bingeing on beer! Actually, it's not. *The Guardian*. Retrieved from http://www.guardian.co.uk/commentisfree/2012/mar/23/beer-britain-liver-disease?INTCMP=ILCNETTXT3487.

Brownson, R.C., Chriqui, J.F., and Stamatakis, K.A. (2009). Understanding evidence-based public health policy. *American Journal of Public Health, 99*(9), 1576–83.

Brugha, R., and Varvasovszky, Z. (2000). Stakeholder analysis: A review. *Health Policy and Planning, 15*(3), 239–46.

Bruun, K. (1971). Alkoholitutkimuksen kolme kulmakiveä (Three cornerstones of alcohol research). *Alkoholikysymys, 39*(2), 32–7.

Bruun, K., Edwards, G., Lumio, M., et al. (1975). *Alcohol Control Policies in Public Health Perspective*. The Finnish Foundation for Alcohol Studies, (vol. 25). New Brunswick, NJ: Rutgers University Center of Alcohol Studies.

Butler, S. (2009). Obstacles to the implementation of an integrated national alcohol policy in Ireland. *Journal of Social Policy, 38*(2), 343–59.

Butterfield, L.H. (1950). The reputation of Benjamin Rush. *Pennsylvania History, 17*(1), 3–22.

Caetano, R., and Laranjeira, R. (2006). A "perfect storm" in developing countries: Economic growth and the alcohol industry. *Addiction, 101*, 149–52.

Cagney, P., and Palmer, S. (2007). *The Sale and Supply of Alcohol to Under 18 Year Olds in New Zealand: A Systematic Overview of International And New Zealand Literature*. Wellington, New Zealand: Research New Zealand. Retrieved from: http://www.justice.govt.nz/publications/global-publications/t/the-sale-and-supply-of-alcohol-to-under-18-year-olds-in-new-zealand-a-systematic-overview-of-International-and-new-zealand-literature-final-report.

Calhoun, F., and Warren, K. (2007). Fetal alcohol syndrome: Historical perspectives. *Neuroscience and Biobehavioral Reviews, 31*, 168–71.

Caplan, N. (1979). The two-communities theory and knowledge utilization. *American Behavioral Scientist, 22*(3), 459–70.

Carcah, C., and James, M. (1998). *Homicide between Intimate Partners in Australia*. Canberra, Australia: Australian Institute of Criminology.

Carrell, S. (2012, 24 May). Scottish Parliament backs cut-price alcohol clampdown. *The Guardian*. Retrieved from http://www.guardian.co.uk/society/2012/may/24/scottish-parliament-cut-price-alcohol-clampdown?newsfeed=true.

Carroll, J. (2007, 27 July). Most Americans oppose lowering legal drinking age to 18 nationwide. *Gallup News Service*. Retrieved from http://www.gallup.com/poll/28237/Most-Americans-Oppose-Lowering-Legal-Drinking-Age-Nationwide.aspx.

Carroll, L. (1976). The temperance movement in India: Politics and social reform. *Modern Asian Studies*, *10*(3), 417–47.

Carroll, L. (2003, 4 November). Alcohol's toll on fetuses: Even worse than thought. *New York Times*. Retrieved from http://www.nytimes.com/2003/11/04/science/alcohol-s-toll-on-fetuses-even-worse-than-thought.html.

Carter, A., Miller, P.G., and Hall, W. (2012). The ethics of harm reduction. In R. Pates and D. Riley (eds), *Harm reduction in substance use and high-risk behavior: International policy and practice* (pp. 111–22). Chichester, UK: Wiley-Blackwell.

Carter, D. (2005, 8 June). Sale of Liquor (Youth Alcohol Harm Reduction) Amendment Bill. New Zealand, Parliament, House of Representatives. *Hansard*, *626*, p. 21163. Retrieved from http://www.parliament.nz/en-NZ/PB/Debates/Debates/d/5/5/47HansD_20050608_00000975-Sale-of-Liquor-Youth-Alcohol-Harm-Reduction.htm.

Center for Science in the Public Interest (n.d.). Fact sheet: Fetal alcohol syndrome. Washington, DC: Author. Retrieved from http://www.cspinet.org/booze/fas.htm.

Centers for Disease Control (CDC) (1994, 2 December). Current trends update: Alcohol-related traffic fatalities—United States, 1982–1993. *Morbidity and Mortality Weekly Report (MMWR)*, *43*(47), 861–3. Retrieved from http://www.cdc.gov/mmwr/preview/mmwrhtml/00033780.htm.

Centers for Disease Control (2006). Alcohol factsheet—general information. Retrieved from http://www.cdc.gov/alcohol/factsheets/general_information.htm.

Centers for Disease Control (2012a). Alcohol and public health: Frequently asked questions. Retrieved from http://www.cdc.gov/alcohol/faqs.htm#standDrink.

Centers for Disease Control (2012b). Deaths: Final data for 2009. *National Vital Statistics Report*, *60*(3). Retrieved from http://www.cdc.gov/nchs/products/nvsr.htm.

Chavkin, W. (1990). Drug addiction and pregnancy: Policy crossroads. *American Journal of Public Health*, *80*(4), 483–7.

Chen, M., Grube, J.W., Nygaard, P., and Miller, B.A. (2008). Identifying social mechanisms for the prevention of adolescent drinking and driving. *Accident Analysis and Prevention*, *40*(2), 576–85.

Children and drink: What's legal? (2007, 27 April). *BBC News*. Retrieved from http://news.bbc.co.uk/1/hi/uk/6598867.stm.

Chisholm, D., Rehm, J., Van Ommeren, M., and Monteiro, M. (2004). Reducing the global burden of hazardous alcohol use: A comparative cost-effectiveness analysis. *Journal of Studies on Alcohol and Drugs, 65*(6), 783–93.

Choi, B.C.K., Pang, T., Lin. V., et al. (2005). Can scientists and policy makers work together? *Journal of Epidemiology and Community Health, 59*(8), 632–7.

Christiansen, B.A., Goldman, M.S., and Inn, A. (1982). Development of alcohol-related expectancies in adolescents: Separating pharmacological from social-learning influences. *Journal of Consulting and Clinical Psychology, 50*(3), 336–44.

Chrzan, J. (2011). Book review of *Breaking the Ashes: The Culture of Illicit Liquor in Sri Lanka* by M.R. Gamburd and *Benelong's Heaven: Recovery from Alcohol and Drug Abuse within an Aboriginal Australian Residential Treatment Center* by R. Chenhall. *Medical Anthropology Quarterly, 25*(1), 122–6.

Chudley, A.E., Conry, J., Cook, J.L., et al. (2005). Fetal alcohol spectrum disorder: Canadian guidelines for diagnosis. *Canadian Medical Association Journal, 172*, S1–S21.

Clark, A. (2010, 16 October). Drunk driving: Is the blood-alcohol limit too liberal? *Time.* Retrieved from http://www.time.com/time/nation/article/0,8599,2025301,00.html.

Clark, A.H., and Foy, D.W. (2000). Trauma exposure and alcohol use in battered women. *Violence Against Women, 6*(1), 37–48.

Clark, P. (1983). *The English Alehouse: A Social History, 1200–1830.* London: Longman Higher Education.

Clarren, S.K. (2009). Time for the development of effective approaches for the prevention of fetal alcohol spectrum disorder? *Expert Review of Obstetrics and Gynecology, 4*(5), 483–5.

Clarren, S.K., and Salmon, A. (2010). Prevention of Fetal Alcohol Spectrum Disorder: Proposal for a comprehensive approach. *Expert Review of Obstetrics and Gynecology, 5*(1), 23–30.

Cocker, B. (1860). *A Plea for the Widow and Orphan against the Traffic in Alcohol.* Chicago, IL: Press and Tribune Book and Job Printing Office.

Cole, M. (2011, 5 January). Mine's a … two-thirds of a pint. *The Guardian.* Retrieved from http://www.guardian.co.uk/commentisfree/2011/jan/05/two-thirds-pint-new-beer-size.

Coleman, W.T. (1984, April). The right move, but the wrong solution. *American Bar Association Journal, 70*, 18–24.

Collins, D., and Lapsley, H. (2008). *The Costs of Tobacco, Alcohol and Illicit Drug Abuse to Australian Society in 2004/05.* Canberra, Australia: Commonwealth Department of Health and Ageing.

Connor, W.D. (1979). Alcohol and Soviet society. In M. Marshall (ed.), *Beliefs, Behaviours, and Alcoholic Beverages: A Cross-Cultural Survey* (pp. 433–50). Ann Arbor, MI: University of Michigan Press.

Conroy, D.W. (1995). *In Public Houses: Drink and The Revolution of Authority in Colonial Massachusetts*. Chapel Hill, NC: The University of North Carolina Press.

Conroy, D.W. (2006). In the public sphere: Efforts to curb the consumption of rum in Connecticut, 1760–1820. In M.P. Holt (ed.), *Alcohol: A Social and Cultural History* (pp. 41–60). Oxford, UK: Berg.

Cook, P.J. (2007). *Paying the Tab: The Costs and Benefits of Alcohol Control*. Princeton, NJ: Princeton University Press.

Cook, P.J. (2010). Leave the minimum drinking age to the states. In N.A. Frost, J.D. Freilich, and T.R. Clear (eds), *Contemporary Issues in Criminal Justice Policy: Policy Proposals from the American Society of Criminology Conference* (pp. 99–106). Belmont, CA: Wadsworth, Cengage Learning.

Cook, P.J., and Gearing, M.E. (2010). The minimum legal drinking age: 21 as an artifact. In H.R. White and D.L. Rabiner (eds), *College Drinking and Drug Use* (pp. 275–93). New York: The Guilford Press.

Cook, P.J., and Tauchen, G. (1984). The effect of minimum drinking age legislation on youthful auto fatalities, 1970–1977. *The Journal of Legal Studies*, *13*(1), 169–90.

Cooper, M. (2011, 19 July). Utah's liquor laws, as mixed up as some drinks. *New York Times*. Retrieved from http://www.nytimes.com/2011/07/20/us/20liquor.html?_r=1&hp.

Coughlan, S. (2006, 17 August). The secret life of the round. *BBC News*. Retrieved from http://news.bbc.co.uk/1/hi/magazine/4798919.stm.

Crampton, R., and Burgess, M. (2009). The price of everything, the value of nothing: A (truly) external review of BERL's study of harmful alcohol and drug use. Working paper No. 10/2009, Department of Economics and Finance, University of Canterbury, Christchurch, New Zealand.

Crawford, I., and Tanner, S. (1995). *Alcohol Taxes and the Single European Market*. London: Institute for Fiscal Studies.

Critcher, C. (2011). Drunken panics: The gin craze, binge drinking and the political economy of moral regulation. In S.P. Hier (ed.), *Moral Panic and the Politics of Anxiety* (pp. 171–89). Abingdon, UK: Routledge.

Culp, R.F. (2005). The rise and stall of prison privatization: An integration of policy analysis perspectives. *Criminal Justice Policy Review, 16*, 412–42.

Daley, S. (2001, 28 March). Europe making Sweden ease alcohol rules. *New York Times*, p. A1. Retrieved from www.proquest.com.

Dalziel, L. (2005, 8 June). Sale of Liquor (Youth Alcohol Harm Reduction) Amendment Bill. New Zealand, Parliament, House of Representatives. *Hansard, 626*, p. 21163. Retrieved from http://www.parliament.nz/en-NZ/PB/Debates/Debates/d/5/5/47HansD_20050608_00000975-Sale-of-Liquor-Youth-Alcohol-Harm-Reduction.htm.

Darialova, N. (1991, 18 February). Vodka: The opiate of the masses. *Forbes, 147*, p. 96–8.

Davies, L. (2005). 25 years of saving lives. *Driven*, Fall 2005. 8–17. Retrieved from http://www.madd.org/about-us/history/madd25thhistory.pdf.

Davies, P., and Walsh, D. (1983). *Alcohol Problems and Alcohol Control in Europe*. New York: Gardner Press.

Davison, L. (1992). Experiments in the social regulation of industry: Gin legislation, 1729–1751. In L. Davison, T. Hitchcock, T. Keirn, and R.B. Shoemaker (eds), *Stilling the Grumbling Hive: The Response to Social And Economic Problems in England, 1689–1750* (pp. 25–48). Stroud, UK: Alan Sutton.

Dawson, D. (2003). Methodological issues in measuring alcohol use. Bethesda, MD: National Institute on Alcohol Abuse and Alcoholism. Retrieved from http://pubs.niaaa.nih.gov/publications/arh27-1/18-29.htm.

de Castella, T. (2012, 21 February). 10 radical solutions to binge drinking. *BBC News Magazine*. Retrieved from http://www.bbc.co.uk/news/magazine-16466646.

de Jong, K., Mulhern, M., Ford, N., et al. (2002). Psychological trauma of the civil war in Sri Lanka. *The Lancet, 359*, 1517–18.

De Mel, N. (2001). Women and the nation's narrative: Gender and nationalism in twentieth century Sri Lanka. Lanham, MD: Rowman and Littlefield.

De Silva, K.M. (1981). *A History of Sri Lanka*. London: C. Hurst and Co.

DeJong, W., and Hingson, R. (1998). Strategies to reduce driving under the influence of alcohol. *Annual Review of Public Health, 19*, 359–78.

Deloria, V., and Wilkins, D.E. (1999). *Tribes, Treaties, and Constitutional Tribulations*. Austin, TX: The University of Texas Press.

Department for Children, Schools and Families, Home Office, and Department of Health (2008). *Youth Alcohol Action Plan*. Norwich, UK: The Stationery Office.

Department for National Drug Control (Bermuda) (n.d.). Treatment and rehabilitation. Retrieved from http://www.gov.bm/portal/server.pt?open=512&objID=663&&PageID=232584&mode=2&in_hi_userid=1.

Department of Health (1992). *The Health of The Nation: A Strategy for Health in England*. Norwich, UK: Her Majesty's Stationery Office.

Department of Health for Hong Kong, Special Administrative Region of China (2011). *Action Plan to Reduce Alcohol-Related Harm in Hong Kong*. Retrieved from http://www.dh.gov.hk/english/pub_rec/pub_rec_ar/pdf/ncd_ap2/action_plan_whole_document_e.pdf.

Dillon, P. (2002). *Gin: The Much Lamented Death of Madam Geneva*. Boston, MA: Justin, Charles & Co.

Dingwall, G. (2007). Responding to alcohol-related crime and disorder in England and Wales: Understanding the government's "blitz." *Security Journal, 20*, 284–92.

Dinh-Zaar, T., Diguiseppi, C., Heitman, E. and Roberts, I. (1999). Preventing injuries through interventions for problem drinking: A systematic review of randomized controlled trials. *Alcohol and Alcoholism, 34*(4), 609–21.

Directorate-General for Health and Consumer Protection (2006). Alcohol-related harm in Europe: Key data. Brussels: Author, European Commission. Retrieved from http://ec.europa.eu/health/archive/ph_determinants/life_style/alcohol/documents/alcohol_factsheet_en.pdf.

Dobbin, F., Simmons, B., and Garrett, G. (2007). The global diffusion of public policies: Social construction, coercion, competition, or learning? *Annual Review of Sociology*, *33*, 449–72.

Dobson, R., and Owen, J. (2012, 13 May). Tests begin on new drink-busting drug. *The Independent*. Retrieved from http://www.independent.co.uk/news/science/tests-begin-on-new-drinkbusting-drug-7742366.html.

Dolowitz, D.P., and Marsh, D. (2000). Learning from abroad: The role of policy transfer in contemporary policy-making. *Governance: An International Journal of Policy and Administration*, *13*(1), 5–24.

Dongier, M. (2003). What treatment options exist for alcohol abuse? *Journal of Psychiatry and Neuroscience*, *28*(1), 80.

Doos, A. (1982, 18 June). $8 for a bar drink: Sweden pressing anti-alcohol drive. *Los Angeles Times*. Retrieved from www.proquest.com.

Douglas, M. (ed.). (1987). *Constructive drinking: Perspectives on Drink from Anthropology*. Cambridge, UK: Cambridge University Press.

Douglass, R., and Freedman, J. (1977). *Alcohol-related Casualties and Alcohol Beverage Market Response to Beverage Alcohol Availability Policies in Michigan*. Ann Arbor, MI: The University of Michigan Highway Safety Research Institute.

Doust, J. (2007, 28 December). Rise of "le binge drinking?" *The Telegraph*. Retrieved from http://www.telegraph.co.uk/expat/4205118/Rise-of-Le-Binge-Drinking.html.

Downie, A. (2006a, 16 February). In Brazil, partial prohibition. *The Christian Science Monitor*. Retrieved from http://www.csmonitor.com/2006/0216/p06s01-woam.html.

Downie, A. (2006b, 1 June). Brazil's new closing time. *Time*. Retrieved from http://www.time.com/time/world/article/0,8599,1199963,00.html.

Drinking age lowered in Michigan. (1972, 4 January). *Chicago Daily Defender*. Retrieved from www.proquest.com.

Drinking age should rise—poll. (2012, 2 July). *Otago Daily Times*. Retrieved from http://www.odt.co.nz/news/national/215279/drinking-age-should-rise-poll.

Duailibi, S., Ponicki, W., Grube, J., et al. (2007). The effect of restricting opening hours on alcohol-related violence. *American Journal of Public Health*, *97*(12), 2276–80.

Dunn, W.N. (1980). The two-communities metaphor and models of knowledge use. *Science Communication*, *1*(4), 515–36.

Edwards, G., Anderson, P., Babor, T.F., et al. (1994). *Alcohol Policy and the Public Good*. Oxford, UK: Oxford University Press.

Elders, C.L. (2007). Variations in ADH and ALDH in Southwest California Indians. *Alcohol Research and Health*, *30*(1), 14–17.

Emmons, B. (2000). *The Book of Gins and Vodkas*. Chicago, IL: Carus Publishing.

Endal, D. (2010). New alcohol policy in the making in Malawi. Retrieved from http://www.add-resources.org/new-alcohol-policy-in-the-making-in-malawi.4819531.html.

Engs, R.C. (1995). Do traditional Western European drinking practices have origins in Antiquity? *Addiction*, *2*(3), 227–39.

Eriksen, S. (2003). Sweden. In J.S. Blocker, D.M. Fahey, and I.R. Tyrrell (eds), *Alcohol and Temperance in Modern History: A Global Encyclopedia* (pp. 603–5). Santa Barbara, CA: ABC-CLIO.

Eurocare (2010, 20 May). Eurocare welcomes the adoption of Global Alcohol Strategy by the WHO. Retrieved from http://www.eurocare.org/library/updates/eurocare_welcomes_the_adoption_of_global_alcohol_strategy_by_the_who.

European Commission (2006). *Communication from the Commission to the Council, the European Parliament, the European Economic and Social Committee and the Committee of the Regions: An EU Strategy to Support Member States in Reducing Alcohol Related Harm*. Brussels, Belgium: Author. Retrieved from http://eur-lex.europa.eu/LexUriserv/site/en/com/2006/com2006_0625en01.pdf.

European Strategy to Reduce Alcohol-Related Harm (2011). Communication from the European Commission, 24 October 2006. Retrieved from http://europa.eu/legislation_summaries/public_health/health_determinants_lifestyle/c11564b_en.htm.

Evans, L. (2004). *Traffic Safety*. Bloomfield Hills, MI: Science Serving Society.

Everitt, R., and Jones, P. (2002). Changing the minimum legal drinking age— Its effect on a central city emergency department. *New Zealand Medical Journal*, *115*(1146), 9–11.

Farrell, M. (1990). News and notes. *British Journal of Addiction*, *85*(3), 427.

Fast, D.K., and Conry, J. (2009). Fetal alcohol spectrum disorders and the criminal justice system. *Development Disabilities Research Reviews*, *15*, 250–57.

Fell, J.C., Fisher, D.A., Voas, R.B., et al. (2009). The impact of underage drinking laws on alcohol-related fatal crashes of young drivers. *Alcoholism: Clinical and Experimental Research*, *33*(7), 1208–19.

Ferdinandis, T.G.H.C. and de Silva, H.J. (2008). Illicit alcohol consumption and neuropathy—A preliminary study in Sri Lanka. *Alcohol and Alcoholism*, *43*(2), 171–3.

Ferentzy, P. (2001). From sin to disease: Differences and similarities between past and current conceptions of chronic drunkenness. *Contemporary Drug Problems*, *28*, 363–90.

Fergusson, D., and Boden, J. (2011). Alcohol use in adolescence. In P.D. Gluckman (ed.), *Improving the Transition: Reducing Social and Psychological Morbidity*

During Adolescence (pp. 235–56). Auckland, New Zealand: Office of the Prime Minister's Science Advisory Committee.

Fernández-Serrano, M.J., Pérez-García, M., Schmidt Río-Valle, J., and Verdejo-García, A. (2010). Neuropsychological consequences of alcohol and drug abuse on different components of executive functions. *Journal of Psychopharmacology*, *24*(9) 1317–32.

Ferri, M., Amato, L., and Davoli, M. (2006). *Alcoholics Anonymous and Other 12-step Programmes for Alcohol Dependence*. The Cochrane Collaboration: Cochrane Drugs and Alcohol Group.

Field, M.G., and Powell, D.E. (1981). Alcohol abuse in the Soviet Union. *The Hastings Center Report*, *11*(5), 40–44.

Figlio, D. (1995). The effect of drinking age laws and alcohol-related crashes: Time-series evidence from Wisconsin. *Journal of Policy Analysis and Management*, *14*(4), 555–66.

Filkins, L.D., and Flora, J.D. (1982). *Alcohol-related Accidents and DUIL Arrests in Michigan: 1978–1980*. Ann Arbor, MI: Transportation Research Institute.

Findlay, R.A., Sheehan, M.C., Davey, J., et al. (2002). Liquor law enforcement: Policy and practice in Australia. *Drugs: Education, Prevention and Policy*, *9*(1), 85–94.

Fleming, G. (2006, 3 May). Keep drinking age at 18, say doctors. *New Zealand Herald*. Retrieved from http://www2.potsdam.edu/hansondj/inthenews/underagedrinking/20060623142230.html.

Florio, J.J. (1984, April). Raise it to 21 and end the carnage. *American Bar Association Journal*, *70*, 18–24.

Ford, D. (2011, 11 October). Diane Sawyer reporting: A hidden America: Children of the plains. *ABC News*. Retrieved from http://abcnews.go.com/blogs/headlines/2011/10/diane-sawyer-reporting-a-hidden-america-children-of-the-plains-on-friday-october-14.

Forsyth, A.J.M. (2008). Banning glassware from nightclubs in Glasgow (Scotland): Observed impacts, compliance and patron's views. *Alcohol and Alcoholism*, *43*(1), 111–17.

Fox, A. (2008). Sociocultural factors that foster or inhibit alcohol-related violence. In *Alcohol and Violence: Exploring Patterns and Response* (pp. 1–28). Washington, DC: International Center for Alcohol Policies.

Fox, K. (2011, 12 October). Viewpoint: Is the alcohol message all wrong? *BBC News*. Retrieved from http://www.bbc.co.uk/news/magazine-15265317.

Frances, A. (2010, 25 March). DSM5 "addiction" swallows substance abuse. *Psychology Today*. Retrieved from http://www.psychologytoday.com/blog/dsm5-in-distress/201003/dsm5-addiction-swallows-substance-abuse.

Frank, J.W., Moore, R.S., and Ames, G.M. (2000). Historical and cultural roots of drinking problems among American Indians. *American Journal of Public Health*, *90*(3), 344–51.

Fried, L.P., Kronmal, R.A., Newman, A.B., et al. (1998). Risk factors for 5-year mortality in older adults: The Cardiovascular Health Study. *The Journal of the American Medical Association, 279*(8), 585–92.

Furr-Holden, C.D., Voas, R.B., Lacey, J., et al. (2011). The prevalence of alcohol use disorders among night-time weekend drivers. *Addiction, 106*, 1251–60.

Gadkari, P. (2012, 27 April). Are beer firms to blame for Native American drink woe? *BBC News*. Retrieved from http://www.bbc.co.uk/news/magazine-17859117.

Gamburd, M.R. (2008). *Breaking the Ashes: The Culture of Illicit Liquor in Sri Lanka*. Ithaca, NY: Cornell University Press.

Giago, T. (2012, 13 May). "Beer sniffing" reporters invade Pine Ridge. *Huffington Post*. Retrieved from http://www.huffingtonpost.com/tim-giago/beer-sniffing-reporters-i_b_1513111.html.

Giddens, A. (1999). Risk and responsibility. *Modern Law Review, 62*(1), 1–10.

Giesbrecht, N. (2000). Roles of commercial interests in alcohol policies: Recent developments in North America. *Addiction, 95*, 581–95.

Giesbrecht, N. (2007). Alcohol policies and public opinion: Five case studies on recent developments in Europe and North America. *Journal of Substance Use, 12*(6), 385–8.

Giesbrecht, N., Ialomiteanu, A., Anglin, L., and Adlaf, E. (2007). Alcohol marketing and retailing: Public opinion and recent policy developments in Canada. *Journal of Substance Use, 12*(6), 389–404.

Giglia, R.C., and Binns, C.W. (2007). Patterns of alcohol intake of pregnant and lactating women in Perth, Australia. *Drug and Alcohol Review, 26*, 493–500.

Ginter. E., and Simko, V. (2009). Alcoholism: Recent advances in epidemiology, biochemistry and genetics. *Bratislavské Lekárske Listy, 110*, 307–11.

Gladwell, M. (2010, 15 and 22 February). Drinking games. *The New Yorker*, pp. 70–76.

Glik, D., Prelip, M., Myerson, A., and Eilers, K. (2008). Fetal alcohol syndrome prevention using community-based narrowcasting campaigns. *Health Promotion Practice, 9*(1), 93–103.

Gold, T. (2012, 15 May). Minimum alcohol pricing? Blame those vomiting girls. *The Guardian*. Retrieved from http://www.guardian.co.uk/commentisfree/2012/may/15/alcohol-price-rise-scotland?newsfeed=true.

Golden, J. (1999). "An argument that goes back to the womb": The demedicalization of fetal alcohol syndrome, 1973–1992. *Journal of Social History, 33*(2), 269–98.

Golden, J. (2000). "A tempest in a cocktail glass": Mothers, alcohol, and television, 1977–1996. *Journal of Health Politics, Policy and Law, 25*(3), 473–98.

Golden, J. (2005). *Message in a Bottle: The Making of Fetal Alcohol Syndrome*. Cambridge, MA: Harvard University Press.

Gordon, R., Harris, F., Mackintosh, A.M., and Moodie, C. (2011). Assessing the cumulative impact of alcohol marketing on young people's drinking: Cross-sectional data findings. *Addiction Research and Theory, 19*(1), 66–75.

Gorgulho, M., and Da Ros, V. (2006). Country report: Alcohol and harm reduction in Brazil. *International Journal of Drug Policy*, *17*, 350–57.

Goss, C.W., Van Bramer, L.D., Gliner, J.A., Pet al. (2008). Increased police patrols for preventing alcohol-impaired driving. *Cochrane Database of Systematic Reviews*, *4*, 1–89.

Gossop, M. (2007). *Living with Drugs* (6th ed.). Aldershot, UK: Ashgate.

Graham, K. (2005). Public drinking then and now. *Contemporary Drug Problems*, *32*, 45–56.

Graham, K., Bernards, S., Wilsnack, S.C., and Gmel, G. (2011). Alcohol may not cause partner violence but it seems to make it worse: A cross national comparison of the relationship between alcohol and severity of partner violence. *Journal of Interpersonal Violence*, *26*(8), 1503–23.

Grant, B.F., Dawson, D.A., Stinson, F.S., et al. (2004). The 12-month prevalence and trends in DSM-IV alcohol abuse and dependence: United States, 1991–1992 and 2001–2002. *Drug and Alcohol Dependence*, *74*(3), 223–34.

Grant, T.M., Ernst, C., Streissguth, A., and Stark, A. (2005). Preventing alcohol and drug exposed births in Washington State: Intervention findings from three Parent-Child Assistance Program sites. *American Journal of Drug and Alcohol Abuse*, *31*(3), 471–90.

Gray, R. (2011). Commentary: Sullivan on the offspring of the female criminal alcoholic. *International Journal of Epidemiology*, *40*, 289–92.

Grayson, D., Saggers, S., Sputore, B., and Bourbon, D. (2000). What works? A review of evaluated alcohol misuse interventions among Aboriginal Australians. *Addiction*, *95*(1), 11–22.

Greenaway, J. (2003). *Drink and British Politics since 1830: A Study in Policy-making*. Basingstoke, UK: Palgrave MacMillan.

Greenfeld, L.A. (1998). *Alcohol and Crime: An Analysis of National Data on the Prevalence of Alcohol Involvement in Crime*. Washington, DC: US Department of Justice, Bureau of Justice Statistics.

Greenfield, T.K., Johnson, S.P., and Giesbrecht, N. (2004). The alcohol policy development process: Policymakers speak. *Contemporary Drug Problems*, *31*, 627–54.

Greenfield, T.K., and Kaskutas, L.A. (1998). Five years' exposure to the alcohol warning label messages and their impacts: Evidence from diffusion analysis. *Applied Behavioral Science Review*, *6*, 39–68.

Greenfield, T.K., Ye, Y., and Giesbrecht, N. (2007). Views of alcohol control policies in the 2000 National Alcohol Survey: What news for alcohol policy development in the US and its states? *Journal of Substance Use*, *12*(6), 429–45.

Group's aim is to outlaw drinking by teens in state. (1977, 24 May). *The Argus-Press*, p. 11.

Gual, A., and Anderson, P. (2012). Introduction. In P. Anderson, F. Braddick, J. Reynolds, and A. Gual (eds), *Alcohol Policy in Europe: Evidence from AMPHORA* (pp. 1–3). Retrieved from: http://amphoraproject.net/view.php?id_cont=45.

Gunasekara, F.I., and Wilson, N. (2010). Very cheap drinking in New Zealand: Some alcohol is more affordable than bottled water and nearly as cheap as milk. *The New Zealand Medical Journal, 123*(1324), 103–7.

Gustafsson, N-K.J. (2010). Changes in alcohol availability, price and alcohol-related problems and the collectivity of drinking cultures: What happened in southern and northern Sweden? *Alcohol and Alcoholism, 45*(5), 456–67.

Gustafsson N-K.J., and Ramstedt, M.R. (2011). Changes in alcohol-related harm in Sweden after increasing alcohol import quotas and a Danish tax decrease: An interrupted time-series analysis for 2000–2007. *International Journal of Epidemiology, 40*, 432–40.

Gustavsson, S. (2007). Reconciling suprastatism and accountability: A view from Sweden. In C. Hoskyns and M. Newman (eds), *Democratizing the European Union: Issues for the Twenty-first Century* (pp. 39–64). New Brunswick, NJ: Transaction Publishers.

Gutting, G. (2012). How reliable are the social sciences? *New York Times* Online Commentary. Retrieved from http://opinionator.blogs.nytimes.com/2012/05/17/how-reliable-are-the-social-sciences.

Habgood, R., Casswell, S., Pledger M., and Bhatt, K. (2001). *Drinking in New Zealand: National Surveys Comparison 1995 and 2000*. Auckland, New Zealand: Alcohol and Public Health Research Unit. Retrieved from http://www.aphru.ac.nz/projects/alcohol%202000%20contents.htm.

Hacker, G.A. (2006, 7 December). Congress Passes Sober Truth on Preventing (STOP) Underage Drinking Act. Center for Science in the Public Interest online posting. Retrieved from http://www.cspinet.org/new/200612071.html.

Hadfield, P., and Newton, A. (2010, September). Alcohol, crime and disorder in the night-time economy. *Factsheet: Alcohol Concern's Information and Statistical Digest*, 1–16.

Haines, L. (2005, 27 March). Study shows drinking age harms teens. *New Zealand Herald*. Retrieved from http://www.nzherald.co.nz/leah-haines/news/article.cfm?a_id=188&objectid=10117304.

Hall, J. (2011, 24 September). "Schooner" lager hits the UK. *The Telegraph*. Retrieved from http://www.telegraph.co.uk/news/uknews/8784563/Schooner-lager-hits-the-UK.html.

Hall, J. (2012, 30 April). A dozen pubs close each week. *The Telegraph*. Retrieved from http://www.telegraph.co.uk/news/uknews/9236865/A-dozen-pubs-close-each-week.html.

Hall, W., and Hunter, E. (1995). Australia. In D.B. Heath (ed.), *International Handbook on Alcohol and Culture* (pp. 7–19). Westport, CT: Greenwood Publishing Group.

Hamm, R.F. (1995). *Shaping the 18th Amendment: Temperance Reform, Legal Culture, and the Polity, 1880–1920*. Chapel Hill, NC: University of North Carolina Press.

Hankin, J.R. (2002). *Fetal Alcohol Syndrome Prevention Research*. Washington, DC: National Institute on Alcohol Abuse and Alcoholism, National Institutes of Health.

Hanson, D.J. (1995). *Preventing Alcohol Abuse: Alcohol, Culture, and Control*. Westport, CT: Greenwood Publishing Group.

Härkönen, J.T., and Mäkelä, P. (2011). Age, period and cohort analysis of light and binge drinking in Finland, 1968–2008. *Alcohol and Alcoholism, 46*(3), 349–56.

Harrell, E. (2009, 29 June). Stemming the rise in global alcohol-related deaths. *Time*. Retrieved from http://www.time.com/time/health/article/0,8599,1907408,00.html.

Harvey, P. (2000). *An Introduction to Buddhist Ethics*. Cambridge, UK: Cambridge University Press.

Harwood, H. (2000). *Updating Estimates of the Economic Costs of Alcohol Abuse in the United States: Estimates, Update Methods, and Data*. Washington, DC: US Department of Health and Human Services, National Institutes of Health, National Institute on Alcohol Abuse and Alcoholism.

Hasin, D., and Keyes, K. (2011). The epidemiology of alcohol and disorders. In B.A. Johnson (ed.), *Addiction Medicine: Science and Practice* (vol. 1) (pp. 23–50). New York: Springer.

Haslam, F. (1996). *From Hogarth to Rowlandson: Medicine in Art in Eighteenth Century Britain*. Liverpool, UK: Liverpool University Press.

Hatton, J., Burton, A., Nash, H., et al. (2009). Drinking patterns, dependency and life-time drinking history in alcohol-related liver disease. *Addiction, 104*(4), 587–92.

Head, B.W. (2008). Three lenses of evidence-based policy. *The Australian Journal of Public Administration, 67*(1), 1–11.

Heath, D.B. (1958). Drinking patterns of the Bolivian Camba. *Quarterly Journal of Studies on Alcohol, 19*(3), 491–508.

Heath, D.B. (1987). Decade of development in the anthropological study of alcohol use: 1970–1980. In M. Douglas (ed.), *Constructive Drinking: Perspectives on Drink from Anthropology* (pp. 16–69). Cambridge, UK: Cambridge University Press.

Heath, D.B. (1995). An anthropological view of alcohol and culture in International perspective. In D.B. Heath (ed.), *International Handbook on Alcohol and Culture* (pp. 328–47). Westport, CT: Greenwood Press.

Henderson, J., Kesmodel, U., and Gray, R. (2007). Systematic review of the fetal effects of prenatal binge-drinking. *Journal of Epidemiology and Community Health, 61*, 1069–73.

Herlihy, P. (2002). *The Alcoholic Empire: Vodka and Politics in Late Imperial Russia*. Oxford, UK: Oxford University Press.

Hernandez-Avila, C.A., and Kranzler, H.R. (2011). Alcohol use disorders. In J.H. Lowinson and P. Ruiz (eds), *Substance Abuse: A Comprehensive Textbook* (5th ed.) (pp. 138–60). Philadelphia, PA: Lippincott Williams & Wilkins.

Híjar, M., Flores, M., López, M.V., and Rosovsky, H. (1998). Alcohol intake and severity of injuries on highways in Mexico: A comparative analysis. *Addiction*, *93*(10), 1543–51.

Hill, L. (2000). The alcohol scene in New Zealand. *The Globe*, *1*, 6–7.

Hill, L., and Stewart, L. (1996). The Sale of Liquor Act, 1989: Reviewing regulatory practices. *Social Policy Journal of New Zealand*, *7*. Retrieved from http://www. msd.govt.nz/about-msd-and-our-work/publications-resources/journals-and-magazines/social-policy-journal/spj07/sale-of-liquor-act.html.

Hingson, R.W., Scotch, N., Mangione, T., et al. (1983). Impact of legislation raising the legal drinking age in Massachusetts from 18 to 20. *American Journal of Public Health*, *73*(2), 163–70.

Hingson, R., Howland, J., Schiavone, T., and Damiata, M. (1990). The Massachusetts Saving Lives Program: Six cities under the focus from drunk driving to speeding, reckless driving and failure to wear safety belts. *Journal of Traffic Medicine*, *3*, 123–32.

Hingson, R., McGovern, T., Howland, J., et al. (1996). Reducing alcohol impaired driving in Massachusetts: The Saving Lives Program. *American Journal of Public Health*, 86, 791–7.

Hinote, B.P., Cockerham, W.C., and Abbott, P. (2009). The specter of post-communism: Women and alcohol in eight post-Soviet states. *Social Science & Medicine*, *68*, 1254–62.

Hirschel, D., Hutchison, I.W., and Shaw, M. (2010). The interrelationship between substance abuse and the likelihood of arrest, conviction, and re-offending in cases of intimate partner violence. *Journal of Family Violence*, *25*, 81–90.

Hoffman, J. (2005, 25 January). Sorting out ambivalence over alcohol and pregnancy. *New York Times*. Retrieved from http://www.nytimes. com/2005/01/25/health/policy/25conv.html?_r=1.

Holder, H., Agardh, E., Högberg, P., et al. (2008). *Alcohol Monopoly and Public Health: Potential Effects of Privatization of the Swedish Alcohol Retail Monopoly*. Stockholm, Sweden: Swedish National Institute of Public Health.

Holt, J.B., Miller, J.W., Naimi, T.S., and Sui, D.Z. (2006). Religious affiliation and alcohol consumption in the United States. *The Geographical Review*, *96*(4), 523–42.

Holt, M. (2006). Europe divided: Wine, beer, and the Reformation in sixteenth-century Europe. In M.P. Holt (ed.), *Alcohol: A Social and Cultural History* (pp. 25–40). Oxford, UK: Berg.

Holtan, N.R. (2002). Partnering helps prevent community alcohol and drug problems. *The Journal for Quality and Participation*, *25*(2), 26–9.

Holzknecht, H. (1996). Policy reform, customary tenure and stakeholder clashes in Papua New Guinea's rainforests. Rural Development Forestry Network Paper 19c. London: Overseas Development Institute.

Homel, R. (1988). Random breath testing in Australia: A complex deterrent. *Australian Drug and Alcohol Review*, *7*, 231–41.

Homel, R. (1990). Crime on the roads: Drinking and driving. In J. Vernon (ed.), *Alcohol and Crime* (pp. 67–82). Canberra, Australia: Australian Institute of Criminology.

Homel, R., and Clark, J. (1994). The prediction and prevention of violence in pubs and clubs. In R.V. Clarke (ed.), *Crime Prevention Studies*, vol. 3. Monsey, NY: Criminal Justice Press.

Hope, A., Gill, A., Costello. G., et al. (2005). *Alcohol and injuries in the Accident and Emergency Department: A national perspective.* Dublin, Ireland: Department of Health and Children.

Hope, C. (2011, 3 January). To halt binge drinking, stop buying rounds. *The Telegraph.* Retrieved from http://www.telegraph.co.uk/health/healthnews/8236863/to-halt-binge-drinking-stop-buying-rounds.html.

How many units is my drink? (2003, 9 December). *BBC News.* Retrieved from http://news.bbc.co.uk/1/hi/uk/3303805.stm.

Huang, W., and Lai, C. (2011). Survival risk factors for fatal injured car and motorcycle drivers in single alcohol-related and alcohol-unrelated vehicle crashes. *Journal of Safety Research, 42*, 93–9.

Hübner, L. (2012). Swedish public opinion on alcohol and alcohol policy, 1995 and 2003. *Journal of Substance Use, 17*(3), 218–29.

Huckle, T., Pledger, M., and Casswell, S. (2006). Trends in alcohol-related harms and offences in a liberalized alcohol environment. *Addiction, 101*(2), 232–40.

Hughes, C.E., and Stevens, A. (2012). A resounding success or a disastrous failure: Re-examining the interpretation of evidence on the Portugese decriminalisation of illicit drugs. *Drug and Alcohol Review, 31*, 101–13.

Humphrys, J. (2010, 17 April). Binge-drinking: What happened to our sense of shame? *The Telegraph.* Retrieved from http://www.telegraph.co.uk/news/uknews/crime/7601915/Binge-drinking-What-happened-to-our-sense-of-shame.html.

Hunter, E., Hall, W., and Spargo, R. (1992). Patterns of alcohol consumption in the Kimberely Aboriginal population. *Medical Journal of Australia, 156*, 764–8.

Hussain, W. (2012, 16 May). Good profit vs. bad profit. *New York Times: Room for Debate.* Retrieved from http://www.nytimes.com/roomfordebate/2012/05/16/how-to-address-alcoholism-on-Indian-reservations/good-profit-vs-bad-profit.

In praise of … the pint. (2011, 7 January). Editorial. *The Guardian.* Retrieved from http://www.guardian.co.uk/commentisfree/2011/jan/07/in-praise-of-the-pint-editorial.

Innvaer, S., Vist, G., Trommald, M., and Oxman, A. (2002). Health policy makers' perceptions of their use of evidence: a systematic review. *Journal of Health Services Research and Policy, 7*(4), 239–44.

Insel, P., Ross, D., McMahon, K., and Bernstein, M. (2013). *Nutrition* (4th ed.). Burlington, MA: Jones & Bartlett Learning.

Institute of Alcohol Studies (2010). *Alcohol Problems, Causes and Prevention.* St Ives, UK: Author. Retrieved from http://www.ias.org.uk/resources/factsheets/problems_causes_prevention.pdf.

International Center for Alcohol Policies (2010a). Blood alcohol concentration (BAC) limits worldwide. Retrieved from http://www.icap.org/Policytools/ICAPIssuesBriefings.

International Center for Alcohol Policies (2010b). International drinking guidelines. Retrieved from http://www.icap.org/PolicyIssues/DrinkingGuidelines/tabid/102/Default.aspx.

Ismail, S., Buckley, S., Budacki, R., et al. (2010). Screening, diagnosing and prevention of fetal alcohol syndrome: Is this syndrome treatable? *Developmental Neuroscience, 32*, 91–100.

James, W. (2008, originally published 1902). *The Varieties of Religious Experience: A Study in Human Nature.* Rockville, MD: ARC Manor.

Jayne, M., Valentine, G., and Holloway, S.L. (2008). Geographies of alcohol, drinking and drunkenness: A review of progress. *Progress in Human Geography, 32*(2), 247–63.

Jayne, M., Valentine, G., and Holloway, S.L. (2010). *Alcohol, Drinking, Drunkenness: (Dis)Orderly Spaces.* Farnham, UK: Ashgate.

Jernigan, D.H., Monteiro, M., Room, R., and Saxena, S. (2000). Towards a global alcohol policy: Alcohol, public health and the role of the WHO. *Bulletin of the World Health Organization, 78*(4), 491–9.

Johnson, H. (2000). The role of alcohol in male partners' assaults on wives. *Journal of Drug Issues, 30*(4), 725–40.

Johnson, K. (2012, 26 May). A taste of prohibition as liquor stores go private. *New York Times.* Retrieved from http://www.nytimes.com/2012/05/27/us/in-washington-state-liquor-stores-are-about-to-go-private.html.

Johnson, S.P., Greenfield, T.K., Giesbrecht, N., et al. (2004). The role of research in the development of U.S. federal alcohol control policy. *Contemporary Drug Problems, 31*, 737–58.

Joksch, H.C., and Jones, R.K. (1993). Changes in the drinking age and crime. *Journal of Criminal Justice, 21*(3), 209–21.

Jones, K.L., Smith, D.W., Ulleland, C.N., and Streissguth, A.P. (1973). Pattern of malformation in the offspring of chronic alcoholic mothers. *Lancet, 1*, 1267–71.

Jones, T., and Newburn, T. (2007). *Policy Transfer in Criminal Justice.* Maidenhead, UK: Open University Press.

Kannangara, A.P. (1984). The riots of 1915 in Sri Lanka: A study in the roots of communal violence. *Past and Present, 102*, 130–65.

Karch, A. (2007). Emerging issues and future directions in state policy diffusion research. *State Politics and Policy Quarterly, 7*(1), 54–80.

Karnani, A.G. (2012, 16 May). Not a private sector problem. *New York Times: Room for Debate.* Retrieved from http://www.nytimes.com/roomfordebate/2012/05/16/how-to-address-alcoholism-on-Indian-reservations/the-reservations-alcoholism-is-not-a-private-sector-problem.

Kasar, M., Gleichgerrcht, E., Keskinkilic, C., et al. (2010). Decision-making in people who relapsed to driving under the influence of alcohol. *Alcoholism: Clinical and Experimental Research, 34*(12), 2162–8.

Kaskutas, L.A. (2008). Letters to the editor: Comments on the Cochrane review on Alcoholics Anonymous effectiveness. *Addiction*, *103*, 1402–3.

Kaskutas, L.A. (2009). Alcoholics Anonymous effectiveness: Faith meets science. *Journal of Addictive Diseases*, *28*(2), 145–57.

Kastor, J. (2010). *The National Institutes of Health, 1991–2008*. Oxford, UK: Oxford University Press.

Katcher, B.S. (1993). Benjamin Rush's educational campaign against hard drinking. *American Journal of Public Health*, *83*(2), 273–81.

Kaysen, D., Simpson, T., Dillworth, T., et al. (2006). Alcohol problems and posttraumatic stress disorder in female crime victims. *Journal of Traumatic Stress*, *19*(3), 399–403.

Kelly, Y.J., Sacker, A., Gray, R., et al. (2012). Light drinking during pregnancy: Still no increased risk for socioemotional difficulties or cognitive deficits at 5 years of age? *Journal of Epidemiology and Community Health*, *66*, 41–8.

Keyser, D.J., Watkins, K.E., Vilamovska, A.-M., and Pincus, H.A. (2008). Improving service delivery for individuals with co-occurring disorders: New perspectives on the quadrant model. *Psychiatric Services*, *59*(11), 1251–3.

Killoran, A., Canning, U., Doyle, N., and Sheppard, L. (2010). *Review of Effectiveness of Laws Limiting Blood Alcohol Concentration Levels to Reduce Alcohol-Related Road Injuries and Deaths*. London: Centre for Public Health Excellence, National Institute for Health and Clinical Excellence.

Kim, J.H., Lee, S., Chow, J., et al. (2008). Prevalence and the factors associated with binge drinking, alcohol abuse, and alcohol dependence: A population-based study of Chinese adults in Hong Kong. *Alcohol and Alcoholism*, *43*(3), 360–70.

Kingdon, J. (2003). *Agendas, Alternatives, and Public Policies* (3rd ed.). New York: Longman.

Kirby, T. (2012). Blunting the legacy of alcohol abuse in Western Australia. *The Lancet*, *379*, 207–8.

Kirley, J. (1978, 13 September). Move to hike drinking age draws debate. *Central Michigan Life*, *60*(7), p. 1.

Klose, K. (1979, 6 December). Alcohol consumption soars in Soviet Union. *Los Angeles Times*, p. D10. Retrieved from www.proquest.com.

Kofoed, L., Friedman, M.J., and Peck, R. (1993). Alcoholism and drug abuse in patients with PTSD. *The Psychiatric Quarterly*, *64*(2), 151–71.

Kondakov, V. (1988, 9 March). Larger vodka lines and casualty lists. *Current Digest of the Soviet Press*, *40*, 16.

König, C., and Segura, L. (2011). Do infrastructures impact on alcohol policy making? *Addiction*, *106*(S1), 47–54.

Kortteinen, T. (ed.) (1989). *State Monopolies and Alcohol Prevention: Report and Working Papers on a Collaborative International Study*. Helsinki, Finland: Social Research Institute on Alcohol Studies, Report 181.

Krasnov, I. (2003). Consumption of alcohol (Russia). In J.S. Blocker, D.M. Fahey, and I.R. Tyrrell (eds), *Alcohol and Temperance in Modern History: A Global Encyclopedia* (pp. 13–16). Santa Barbara, CA: ABC-CLIO.

Krehbiel, K. (1998). *Pivotal Politics: A Theory of US Lawmaking*. Chicago, IL: University of Chicago Press.

Kristof, N.D. (2012a, 6 May). A battle with the brewers. *New York Times*, p. SR13. Retrieved from http://www.nytimes.com/2012/05/06/opinion/sunday/kristof-a-battle-with-the-brewers.html.

Kristof, N.D. (2012b, 10 May). Life is both bleak and brave at Pine Ridge. *Anchorage Daily News*. Retrieved from http://www.adn.com/2012/05/10/2460345/nicholas-kristof-life-is-both.html.

Krulewitch, C.J. (2005). Alcohol consumption during pregnancy. *Annual Review of Nursing Research*, *23*, 101–34.

Kurzer, P. (2001). *Markets and Moral Regulation: Cultural Change in the European Union*. Cambridge, UK: Cambridge University Press.

Kypri, K., Voas, R.B., Langley, J.D., et al. (2006). Minimum purchasing age for alcohol and traffic crash injuries among 15-to-19-Year-Olds in New Zealand. *American Journal of Public Health*, *96*(1), 126–31.

LaChausse, R.G. (2008). The effectiveness of a multimedia program to prevent fetal alcohol syndrome. *Health Promotion Practice*, *9*(3), 289–93.

LaMere, F. (2012, 16 May). Blood on their hands. *New York Times: Room for Debate*. Retrieved from http://www.nytimes.com/roomfordebate/2012/05/16/how-to-address-alcoholism-on-Indian-reservations/nebraska-and-anheuser-busch-caused-the-disaster-at-pine-ridge-and-whiteclay.

Lash, B. (2005). *Young People and Alcohol: Some Statistics to 2003 and 2004 on Possible Effects of Lowering the Purchase Age*. Wellington, New Zealand: Ministry of Justice. Retrieved from http://www.justice.govt.nz/publications/global-publications/y/young-people-and-alcohol-some-statistics-to-2003-and-2004-on-possible-effects-of-lowering-the-purchase-age.

Lasswell, H.D. (1951). The policy orientation. In D. Lerner and H.D. Lasswell (eds), *The Policy Sciences: Recent Developments in Scope and Method*. Palo Alto, CA: Stanford University Press.

Legge, J.S. (1991). *Traffic safety reform in the United States and Great Britain*. Pittsburgh, PA: University of Pittsburgh Press.

Leino, E.V., Romlesjö, A., Shoemaker, C., et al. (1998). Alcohol consumption and mortality II. Studies of male populations. *Addiction*, *93*(2), 205–18.

Leonard, K.E., and Quigley, B.M. (1999). Drinking and marital aggression in newlyweds: An event-based analysis of drinking and the occurrence of husband marital aggression. *Journal of Studies on Alcohol*, *60*, 537–45.

Le Strat, Y., Ramoz, N., Schumann, G., and Gorwood, P. (2008). Molecular genetics of alcohol dependence and related endophenotypes. *Current Genomics*, *9*, 444–51.

Lees, F.R. (1864). *The Condensed Argument for the Legislative Prohibition of the Liquor Traffic*. London: J. Caldwell.

Leonard, K.E. (2008). The role of drinking patterns and acute intoxication in violent interpersonal behaviors. In *Alcohol and Violence: Exploring Patterns and Response* (pp. 29–56). Washington, DC: International Center for Alcohol Policies.

Lerner, B.H. (2011). *One for the Road: Drunk Driving since 1900*. Baltimore, MD: The Johns Hopkins University Press.

Lesch, O.M., Walter, H., Wetschka, C., et al. (2011). *Alcohol and Tobacco: Medical and Sociological Aspects of Use, Abuse and Addiction*. Vienna, Austria: Springer-Verlag.

Levine, H.G. (1993). Temperance cultures: Alcohol as a problem in Nordic and English-Speaking Cultures. In M. Lader, G. Edwards, and D.C. Drummon (eds), *The Nature of Alcohol and Drug-related Problems* (pp. 16–36). New York: Oxford University Press.

Levintova, M. (2007). Russian alcohol policy in the making. *Alcohol and Alcoholism*, *42*(5), 500–505.

Li, G. (2010). Airline accidents. In G. Fink (ed.), *Stress of War, Conflict and Disaster* (pp. 731–4). San Diego, CA: Academic Press.

Lindblom, C.E. (1959). The science of "muddling through." *Public Administration Review*, *19*, 79–88.

Lindblom, C.E. (1979). Still muddling, not yet through. *Public Administration Review*, *39*(6), 517–26.

Liquor consumption falls in Sri Lanka, government says. (2009, 22 September). *Colombo Times*. Retrieved from www.proquest.com.

Litt, J., and McNeil, M. (1997). Biological markers and social differentiation: Crack babies and the construction of the dangerous mother. *Health Care for Women International*, *18*(1), 31–41.

The Liver Centre (2003). Alcohol use. Queensland, Australia: Author. Retrieved from http://www.thelivercentre.com.au/liver-centre/alcoholic-liver-disease.php.

Ljungmark, L. (1979). *Swedish Exodus* (K.B. Westerberg, trans.). Carbondale, IL: Southern Illinois University Press.

London Metropolitan Archives (1998). *Information Leaflet No 3: Licensed Victuallers Records*. London: Author. Retrieved from http://www.cityoflondon. gov.uk/NR/rdonlyres/C03B7200-993B-42B5-8AA6-F5D666D928B9/0/ licensed_victuallers.PDF.

Lönnroth, K., Williams, B., Stadlin, S., et al. (2008). Alcohol use as a risk factor for tuberculosis: A systematic review. *BMC Public Health*, *8*, 289.

Luarkie, R. (2012, 16 May). Communities must be proactive. *New York Times: Room for Debate*. Retrieved from http://www.nytimes.com/roomfordebate/ 2012/05/16/how-to-address-alcoholism-on-Indian-reservations/communities-must-be-proactive-in-addressing-alcoholism-on-reservations.

Lyall, S. (2003, 21 October). Sweden grappling with "alcohol tourism." *The Globe and Mail*, p. A18. Retrieved from www.proquest.com.

Mackinnon, D.P. (1995). Review of the effects of the alcohol warning label. In R.R. Watson (ed.), *Alcohol, Cocaine, and Accidents: Drug and Alcohol Abuse Reviews* (vol. 7) (pp. 131–61). Totowa, NJ: Humana Press.

MacLean, S. (2011). Book review of *Alcohol, Drinking, Drunkenness: (Dis)Orderly Spaces* by M. Jayne, G. Valentine, and S.L. Holloway. *Drug and Alcohol Review, 30*, 689–92.

Magnusson, P., Jakobsson, L., and Hultman, S. (2011). Alcohol interlock systems in Sweden: 10 years of systematic work. *American Journal of Preventive Medicine, 40*(3), 378–9.

Mahal, A. (2000). What works in alcohol policy? Evidence from rural India. *Economic and Political Weekly, 35*(45), 3959–68.

Majzner, M. (2008, 6 June). Swedish alcohol monopoly down the hatch. *The Local*. Retrieved from http://www.thelocal.se/12274/20080606.

Mäkelä, P., and Osterberg, E. (2009). Weakening of one more alcohol control pillar: A review of the effects of the alcohol tax cuts in Finland in 2004. *Addiction, 104*, 554–63.

Males, M. (1986). The minimum purchase age for alcohol and young-driver fatal crashes: A long-term view. *The Journal of Legal Studies, 15*(1), 181–3.

Manning, C. (2011, 18 August). Pubs to sell beer by the schooner. *Mirror*. Retrieved from http://www.mirror.co.uk/money/city-news/pubs-to-sell-beer-by-the-schooner-148084.

Manso, B.P., Faria, M., and Gall, N. (2005). Diadema: Democracy 3: Frontier violence and civilization in São Paulo's periphery. *Braudel Papers*, 36, 3–16.

Manzi, J. (2012). *Uncontrolled: The Surprising Payoff of Trial-And-Error for Business, Politics, and Society*. New York: Basic Books.

Marlatt, G.A., and Witkiewitz, K. (2002). Harm reduction approaches to alcohol use: Health promotion, prevention, and treatment. *Addictive Behaviors, 27*, 867–86.

Marmot, M.G. (2004). Evidence based policy or policy based evidence? *BMJ, 328*, 906–7.

Marriott-Lloyd, P., and Webb, M. (2002). *Tackling Alcohol-Related Offences and Disorder in New Zealand*. Retrieved from http://www.ndp.govt.nz/moh.nsf/0/55A657CFF8203066CC2572F10001B35A.

Marteau, D. (2008). How alcohol may precipitate violent crime. *Drugs and Alcohol Today, 8*(2), 12–16.

Martin, C. R, (2008). The role and value of Alcoholics Anonymous. In C.R. Martin (ed.), *Identification and Treatment of Alcohol Dependency* (pp. 209–14). Keswick, U.K: M&K Update Ltd.

Matsumoto, D. (2007). Culture, context, and behavior. *Journal of Personality, 75*(6), 1285–320.

May, P.A., Fiorentino, D., Coriale, G., et al. (2011). Prevalence of children with severe fetal alcohol spectrum disorders in communities near Rome, Italy: New estimated rates are higher than previous estimates. *International Journal of Environmental Research and Public Health, 8*, 2331–51.

May, P. (1977). Alcohol beverage control: A survey of tribal alcohol statutes. *American Indian Law Review, 5*, 217–28.

May, P.A., and Gossage, J.P. (2001). Estimating the prevalence of fetal alcohol syndrome: A summary. *Alcohol Health*, *25*, 159–67.

May, P.A., Miller, J.H., Goodhart, K.A., et al. (2008). Enhanced case management to prevent fetal alcohol spectrum disorders in Northern Plains communities. *Maternal and Child Health Journal*, *12*(6), 747–59.

McCarthy, J.D., and Wolfson, M. (1996). Resource mobilization by local social movement organizations: Agency, strategy, and organization. *American Sociological Review*, *61*(6), 1070–88.

McConnell, D. (2006, 20 August). Binge drinking is "caused by Irish rounds culture." *Independent*. Retrieved from http://www.independent.ie/national-news/binge-drinking-is-caused-by-irish-rounds-culture-133868.html.

McEwan, B., Campbell, M., and Swain, D. (2010). New Zealand culture of intoxication: Local and global influences. *New Zealand Sociology*, *25*, 15–37.

McFarland, B.H., Gabriel, R.M., Bigelow, D.A., and Walker, R.D. (2006). Organization and financing of alcohol and substance abuse programs for American Indians and Alaska Natives. *American Journal of Public Health*, *96*(8), 1469–77.

McIvor, G., and Tucker, E. (1997, 5 March). Sweden's alcohol monopoly ruled illegal. *Financial Times*, p. 1. Retrieved from www.proquest.com.

McNeal, R.H. (1990). *Stalin: Man and Ruler*. New York: New York University Press.

McSmith, A. (2010, 12 August). First Obama, now Cameron embraces "nudge theory." *Independent*. Retrieved from http://www.independent.co.uk/news/uk/politics/first-obama-now-cameron-embraces-nudge-theory-2050127.html.

McTighe, M.J. (1994). *A Measure of Success: Protestants and Public Culture in Antebellum Cleveland*. Albany, NY: State University of New York Press.

Mears, D.P. (2003). Research and interventions to reduce domestic violence revictimization. *Trauma, Violence, and Abuse*, *4*(2), 127–47.

Media can make great change in society—Thera. (2011, 15 October). *Daily News*. Retrieved from www.proquest.com.

Melecki, S. (2009, 3 February). Nebraska must fight alcoholism on Pine Ridge Reservation. *Daily Nebraskan*. Retrieved from http://www.dailynebraskan.com/opinion/nebraska-must-fight-alcoholism-on-pine-ridge-reservation-1.1353382.

Mendelson, R. (2009). *From Demon to Darling: A Legal History of Wine in America*. Berkeley, CA: University of California Press.

Mercer, S.L., Sleet, D.A., Elder, R.W., et al. (2010). Translating evidence into policy: Lessons learned from the case of lowering the legal blood alcohol limit for drivers. *Annals of Epidemiology*, *20*(6), 412–20.

Mersy, D.J. (2003). Recognition of alcohol and substance abuse. *American Family Physician*, *67*(7), 1529–32.

Miguez-Burbano, M.J. and Jackson, J. (2005). Alcohol and public health. *The Lancet*, *365*(9468), 1386–7.

Miller, P.G., de Groot, F., McKenzie, S., and Droste, N. (2011). Vested interests in addiction research and policy: Alcohol industry use of social aspect public relations organizations against preventative health measures. *Addiction*, *106*, 1560–67.

Miron, J.A., and Tetelbaum, E. (2009a, 15 April). The dangers of the drinking age. *Forbes.com* commentary. Retrieved from http://www.forbes.com/2009/04/15/lowering-legal-drinking-age-opinions-contributors-regulation.html.

Miron, J.A., and Tetelbaum, E. (2009b). Does the Minimum. Legal Drinking Age save lives? *Economic Inquiry*, *47*(2), 317–36.

Miron, J.A., and Zwiebel, J. (1991). Alcohol consumption during Prohibition. Working Paper No. 3675. Cambridge, MA: National Bureau of Economic Research.

Mittelman, A. (2008). *Brewing Battles: A History of American Beer*. New York, NY: Algora Publishing.

Monaghan, M. (2011). *Evidence Versus Politics: Exploiting Research in UK Drug Policy Making?* Bristol, UK: University of Bristol, The Policy Press.

Montag, M. (2012, 18 May). Crime watch: Local activist calls for end to alcohol sales at Whiteclay. *Sioux City Journal*. Retrieved from http://siouxcityjournal.com/blogs/crime_watch/crime-watch-local-activist-calls-for-end-to-alcohol-sales/article_7a9ab0db-660e-595b-a5f4–96e42ab9b92b.html.

Monteiro, M.G. (2007). *Alcohol and Public Health in the Americas: A Case for Action*. Washington, DC: Pan American Health Organization. Retrieved from http://www.who.int/substance_abuse/publications/alcohol_public_health_americas.pdf.

Moreira, T. de C., Ferigolo, M., Fernandes, S., et al. (2011). Alcohol and domestic violence: A cross-over study in residences of individuals in Brazil. *Journal of Family Violence*, *26*, 465–71.

Morone, J.A. (2003). *Hellfire Nation: The Politics of Sin in American History*. New Haven, CT: Yale University Press.

Mosher, J.F., and Jernigan, D.H. (1989). New directions in alcohol policy. *Annual Review of Public Health*, *10*, 245–79.

Mothers Against Drunk Driving (MADD) (1994). *Mothers Against Drunk Driving: Executive Summary of 1993 Results*. Princeton, NJ: Gallup Organization.

MADD (2011). Ignition interlocks: Every state, for every convicted drunk driver. Washington, DC: Author. Retrieved from http://www.madd.org/laws/law-overview/Draft-Ignition_interlocks_Overview.pdf.

MADD (2012). History of the 21 minimum drinking age. Retrieved from http://www.madd.org/underage-drinking/why21/history.html.

MADD milestones: 25 years of making a difference. (2005, Fall). *Driven*, p. 4–7. Retrieved from http://www.madd.org/about-us/history/madd-milestones.pdf.

Mcintosh. J.R. (2003). Gin craze. In J.S. Blocker, D.M. Fahey, and I.R. Tyrrell (eds), *Alcohol and Temperance in Modern History: A Global Encyclopedia* (pp. 265–7). Santa Barbara, CA: ABC-CLIO.

Müller, R. (2004). Introduction: 100 years later—alcohol policies revisited. In R. Müller and H. Klingemann (eds), *From Science to Action? 100 Years Later—Alcohol Policies Revisited* (pp. 1–4). Dordrecht, the Netherlands: Kluwer Academic Publishers.

Mulley, J. (2004). Alcohol in 2004: Why are we pulling in different directions?: RIPH Symposium Wednesday 10 November 2004, London. *Health and Hygiene*, *25*(4), 5–6.

NHS Greater Glasgow and Clyde (2012). Alcohol brief intervention. Retrieved from http://www.nhsggc.org.uk/content/default.asp?page=s1736_2.

National Highway Traffic Safety Administration (2006). *Traffic Safety Facts 2004*. Washington, DC: Author, US Department of Transportation. Retrieved from http://www-nrd.nhtsa.dot.gov/Pubs/TSF2004.pdf.

National Highway Traffic Safety Administration (2007, December). Fatality analysis reporting system (FARS). Retrieved from http://www-fars.nhtsa.dot. gov/Main/index.aspx.

National Highway Traffic Safety Administration (2011, December). *2010 Motor Vehicle Crashes: Overview.* Traffic safety facts research note. Washington, DC: Author.

National Institute for Health and Welfare (Finland) (2012). HiAP and alcohol policies. Retrieved from http://www.thl.fi/en_US/web/en/topics/information_ packages/hiap/hiap-and-alcohol-policies.

National Institute on Alcohol Abuse and Alcoholism (n.d.). Alcohol-related traffic deaths. Retrieved from http://pubs.niaaa.nih.gov/publications/arh27-1/18-29. htm.

National Institute on Alcohol Abuse and Alcoholism (2007, April). Alcohol metabolism: An update. *Alcohol Alert*, *72*, 1–6. Retrieved from http://pubs. niaaa.nih.gov/publications/AA72/AA72.pdf.

Navarro, H.J., Doran, C.M., and Shakeshaft, A.P. (2011). Measuring costs of alcohol harm to others: A review of the literature. *Drug and Alcohol Dependence*, *114*, 87–99.

Nebehay, S. (2010, 20 May). WHO to tackle alcohol misuse, binge drinking (Update 3). Reuters. Retrieved from http://www.reuters.com/ article/2010/05/20/health-alcohol-idUSLDE64J0LN20100520.

Nelson, J.P. (2010). Alcohol, unemployment rates and advertising bans: International panel evidence, 1975–2000. *Journal of Public Affairs*, *10*, 74–87.

Nemtsov, A. (2011). *A Contemporary History of Alcohol in Russia* (H.M. Goldfinger and A. Stickley, trans.). Stockholm. Sweden: Sodertorns hogskola.

New legislation in Sri Lanka. (2006, 29 September). Alcohol, Drugs and Development. Retrieved from http://www.add-resources.org/new-legislation-in-sri-lanka.442468-76602.html.

Newman, T. (2012, 8 May). Alcohol prohibition not helping Native Americans deal with harms of alcohol. *Huffington Post*. Retrieved from http://www. huffingtonpost.com/tony-newman/alcohol-prohibition-not-h_b_1500462. html.

Nicholls, J. (2010). *The Politics of Alcohol: A History of the Drink Question in England*. Manchester, UK: Manchester University Press.

Nicholls, J. (2012, 13 March). How Britain shunned the pub and became a nation of wine drinkers. *The Atlantic*. Retrieved from http://www.theatlantic.com/health/archive/2012/03/how-britain-shunned-the-pub-and-became-a-nation-of-wine-drinkers/254209.

Nochajski, T.H., and Stasiewicz, P.R. (2005). Relapse to driving under the influence (DUI): A review. *Clinical Psychology Review*, *26*(2), 179–95.

Nordlund, S. (2007). The influence of EU on alcohol policy in a non-EU country. *Journal of Substance Use*, *12*(6), 405–18.

Norström, T. (2011). Alcohol and homicide in the United States: Is the link dependent on wetness? *Drug and Alcohol Review*, *30*, 458–65.

Norström, T., Miller, T., Holder, H., et al. (2010). Potential consequences of replacing a retail alcohol monopoly with a private licence system: Results from Sweden. *Addiction*, *105*(12), 2113–19.

Nudge theory of social change is "no silver bullet." (2010, 9 November). *BBC News*. Retrieved from http://www.bbc.co.uk/news/uk-politics-11721155.

Nudge theory trials "are working" say officials. (2012, 8 February). *BBC News*. Retrieved from http://www.bbc.co.uk/news/uk-politics-16943729.

Nutt, D. (2012). *Drugs—Without the Hot Air: Minimising the Harms of Legal and Illegal Drugs*. Cambridge, UK: UIT Cambridge.

Nycander, S. (1998). Ivan Bratt: The man who saved Sweden from Prohibition. *Addiction*, *93*(1), 17–25.

Obot, I.S. (2000). The measurement of drinking patterns and alcohol problems in Nigeria. *Journal of Substance Abuse*, *12*(1/2), 169–81.

O'Farrell, T.J., and Fals-Stewart, W. (2003). *Journal of Marital and Family Therapy*, *29*(1), 121–46.

Office of Justice Programs (2000). *Promising Strategies to Reduce Substance Abuse*. Washington DC: US Department of Justice, Office of Justice Programs.

Oglala Sioux Tribe (2012). South Dakota Department of tourism informational page. Retrieved from http://www.travelsd.com/About-SD/Our-History/Plains-Indians/Sioux-Tribes/Oglala-Sioux-Tribe.

Oglala Sioux Tribe Department of Public Safety (2010). Statement of Chief of Police Richard Greenwald before the U.S. House of Representatives. Retrieved from http://www.ostdps.org.

Ohito, D. (2012, 17 May). Cabinet approves stern traffic rules. *Standard Digital*. Retrieved from http://www.standardmedia.co.ke/?articleID=2000058344&story_title=Cabinet%20approves%20stern%20traffic%20rules.

Oldenburg, R. (1997). *The Great Good Place: Cafés, Coffee Shops, Community Centers, Beauty Parlors, General Stores, Bars, Hangouts, and How They Get You Through The Day*. New York: Marlowe and Company.

Oldenburg, R. (2001). *Celebrating the Third Place: Inspiring Stories About the "Great Good Places" at the Heart of our Communities*. New York: Marlowe and Company.

Oldstone-Moore, J. (2003). Buddhism. In J.S. Blocker, D.M. Fahey, and I.R. Tyrrell (eds), *Alcohol and Temperance in Modern History: A Global Encyclopedia* (pp. 120–21). Santa Barbara, CA: ABC-CLIO.

O'Leary, C.M., Nassar, N., Kurinczuk, J.J., et al. (2010). Prenatal alcohol exposure and risk of birth defects. *Pediatrics*, *126*(4), e843-e850.

O'Neill, I. (2006, 14 August). Scots urged not to buy rounds of drinks. *The Publican's Morning Advertiser*. Retrieved from http://www.morningadvertiser.co.uk/General-News/Scots-urged-not-to-buy-rounds-of-drinks.

Örnberg, J.C. (2013). Alcohol policy in the European Union. In S.L. Greer and P. Kurzer (eds), *European Union Public Health Policy: Regional and Global Trends* (pp. 168–80). Abingdon, UK: Routledge.

Osokina, E.A. (2001, original Russian text published 1999). *Our Daily Bread: Socialist Distribution and the Art of Survival in Stalin's Russia, 1927–1941* (K. Transchel, ed., and K. Transchel and G. Bucher, trans.). Armonk, NY: M.E. Sharpe, Inc.

Österberg, E. (2007). Finnish attitudes to alcohol policy in 2005. *Journal of Substance Use*, *12*(6), 447–60.

Österberg, E., and Karlsson, T. (2002). Studying alcohol policies in national and historical perspectives. In E. Österberg and T. Karlsson (eds), *Alcohol Policies in EU Member States and Norway: A Collection of Country Reports* (pp. 17–42). Helsinki, Finland: STAKES.

Pacific Institute for Research and Evaluation. (2004). *Prevention of Murders in Diadema, Brazil: The Influence of New Alcohol Policies*. Calverton, MD: Author.

Panda, P.K. (2003). *Rights-based Strategies in the Prevention of Domestic Violence*. Washington, DC: International Center for Research on Women.

Parry, C.D.H. (2005). South Africa: Alcohol today. *Addiction*, *100*, 426–9.

Parsons, W. (2002). From muddling through to muddling up: Evidence based policy-making and the modernisation of British government. *Public Policy and Administration*, *17*(3), 43–60.

Partanen, J. (1993). Failures in alcohol policy: Lessons from Russia, Kenya, Truk and history. *Addiction*, 88(Supplement), 129S–34S.

Pathmeshwaran, A. (1997). *The Pattern and Problems of Alcohol Use in Gampaha District*. MD thesis, University of Colombo, Sri Lanka: 2–72.

Paulson, R. (1993). *Hogarth: Art and Politics, 1750–1764*. Cambridge, UK: The Lutterworth Press.

Peadon, E., Payne, J., Henley, N., et al. (2010). Women's knowledge and attitudes regarding alcohol consumption in pregnancy: A national survey. *BMC Public Health*, *10*, 510.

Pechansky, F., and Chandran, A. (2012). Why don't northern American solutions to drinking and driving work in southern America? *Addiction*, *107*(7), 1201–6.

Peck, G. (2009). *The Prohibition Hangover: Alcohol in America from Demon Rum to Cult Cabernet*. Piscataway, NJ: Rutgers University Press.

Pedersen, E., Neighbors, C., and Larimer, M.E. (2010). Differential alcohol expectancies based on type of alcoholic beverage consumed. *Journal of Studies on Alcohol and Drugs*, 925–9.

Peebles, P. (2006). *The History of Sri Lanka*. Westport, CT: Greenwood Publishing Group.

Pelling, R. (2011, 4 January). I'd rather be bankrupt than fail to stump up for my round. *The Telegraph*. Retrieved from http://www.telegraph.co.uk/comment/columnists/rowanpelling/8239794/Id-rather-be-bankrupt-than-fail-to-stump-up-for-my-round.html.

Perera, B., and Torabi, M. (2009). Motivations for alcohol use among men aged 16–30 years in Sri Lanka. *International Journal of Environmental Research and Public Health*, 6, 2408–16.

Pérez, R.L. (2000). Fiesta as tradition, fiesta as change: Ritual, alcohol and violence in a Mexican community. *Addiction*, *95*(3), 365–73.

Perkins, J.J., Sanson-Fisher, R.W., Blunden, S., et al. (1994). The prevalence of drug use in urban Aboriginal communities. *Addiction*, *89*, 1319–31.

Pernanen, K. (2001). Consequences of drinking to friends and the close social environment. In H. Klingemann and G. Gmel (eds), *Mapping the Social Consequences of Alcohol Consumption* (pp. 53–66). Dordrecht, the Netherlands: Kluwer Academic Publishers.

Petrie, D., Doran, C., and Shakeshaft, A. (2011). Willingness to pay to reduce alcohol-related harm in Australian rural communities. *Expert Review of Pharmacoeconomics and Outcomes Research*, *11*(3), 351–63.

Phillips, R. (2003). Gin. In J.S. Blocker, D.M. Fahey, and I.R. Tyrrell (eds), *Alcohol and Temperance in Modern History: A Global Encyclopedia* (pp. 263–5). Santa Barbara, CA: ABC-CLIO.

Poe, Rep. Ted. [TX]. (2007, June 20). Binge drinking and legal age. In *Congressional Record*, vol. *153*(100), pt. 12, p. 16752.

Pompili, M., Serafini, G., Innamorati, M., et al. (2010). Suicidal Behavior and Alcohol Abuse. *International Journal of Environmental Research and Public Health*, *7*(4), 1392–431.

Porter, R. (1985). The drinking man's disease: The "pre-history" of alcoholism in Georgian Britain. *British Journal of Addiction*, *80*(4), 385–96.

Pöschl, G., and Seitz, H.K. (2004). Alcohol and cancer. *Alcohol and Alcoholism*, *39*, 155–65.

Prescott, C.A. (2003). Sex differences in the genetic risk for alcoholism. Bethesda, MD: National Institute on Alcohol Abuse and Alcoholism (NIAAA). Retrieved from: http://www.niaaa.nih.gov/publications/arh26-4/264-273.htm.

Prime Minister's Strategy Unit. (2004). *Alcohol Harm Reduction Strategy for England*. Retrieved from http://www.newcastle-staffs.gov.uk/documents/community%20and%20living/community%20safety/caboffce%20alcoholhar%20pdf.pdf.

Privatizing Sweden's retail alcohol sales will increase alcohol related violence and other harms. (2010, 19 September). *NewsRx Health and Science*, p. 134.

Prohibition, Soviet style. (1990, 15 July). *Richmond Times-Dispatch*, p. C6. Retrieved from www.newsbank.com.

Rahman, F. (2012, 28 April). A better alcohol policy to save lives. *The Malaysian Insider*. Retrieved from http://www.themalaysianinsider.com/opinion/article/a-better-alcohol-policy-to-save-lives.

Ramstedt, M. (2002). Alcohol-related mortality in 15 European countries in the postwar period. *European Journal of Population*, *18*, 307–23.

Reducing homicide in Diadema, Brazil. (n.d.). Cummington, MA: Global Violence Prevention.   Retrieved from http://www.who.int/violenceprevention/about/participants/Homicide.pdf.

Rehm, J., Chisholm, D., Room, R., and Lopez, A.D. (2006a). Alcohol. In D.T. Jamison, J.G. Breman, A.R. Measham, G. Alleyne, et al. (eds), *Disease Control Priorities in Developing Countries* (2nd ed.) (pp. 887–906). Washington, DC: The World Bank.

Rehm, J., Mathers, C., Popova, S., et al. (2009). Global burden of disease and injury and economic cost attributable to alcohol use and alcohol-use disorders. *The Lancet*, *373*(9682), 2223–33.

Rehm, J., Patra, J., Baliunas, D., et al. (2006b). *Alcohol Consumption and the Global Burden of Disease 2002*. Geneva, Switzerland: World Health Organization, Department of Mental Health and Substance Abuse, Management of Substance Abuse.

Rehm, J., Rehn, N., Room, R., et al. (2003). The global distribution of average volume of alcohol consumption and patterns of drinking. *European Addiction Research*, *9*, 147–56.

Rehm, J., Room, R., van den Brink, W. and Jacobi, F. (2005). Alcohol use disorders in EU countries and Norway: An overview of the epidemiology. *European Neuropsychopharmacology*, *15*, 377–88.

Rehn, N., Room, R., and Edwards, G. (2001). *Alcohol in the European Region: Consumption, Harm and Policies*. Copenhagen, Denmark: WHO Regional Office for Europe.

Reid, C. (2012). Cycling and the law. Retrieved from http://www.bikehub.co.uk/featured-articles/cycling-and-the-law.

Rich, R.F. (1991). Knowledge creation, diffusion, and utilization: Perspectives of the Founding Editor of *Knowledge*. *Science Communication*, *12*(3), 319–37.

Richardson, A., and Budd, T. (2003). *Alcohol, Crime and Disorder: A Study of Young Adults*. London: Home Office. Retrieved from http://www.drugsandalcohol.ie/5423/1/Home_office_research_study_263_alcohol,_crime_and_disorder.pdf.

Rigid temperance laws being eased in Sweden. (1967, 15 May). *Washington Post*, p. B5. Retrieved from www.proquest.com.

Riley, E.P., Infante, M.A., and Warren, K.R. (2011). Fetal alcohol spectrum disorders: An overview. *Neuropsychological Review*, *21*, 73–80.

Ritter, A. (2007). Comparing alcohol policies between countries: Science or silliness? *PLoS Medicine*, *4*(4), e153.

Ritter, A., and Bammer, G. (2010). Models of policy-making and their relevance for drug research. *Drug and Alcohol Review, 29,* 352–7.

Robin. G.D. (1991). *Waging the Battle against Drunk Driving: Issues, Countermeasures, and Effectiveness.* Westport, CT: Greenwood Press.

Rodin, A.E. (1981). Infants and gin mania in 18th-century London. *Journal of the American Medical Association, 245*(12), 1237–9.

Rogers, J.D. (1989). Cultural nationalism and social reform: The 1904 Temperance Movement in Sri Lanka. *The Indian Economic and Social History Review, 26*(3), 219–41.

Rohrer, F. (2008, 24 January). Getting your round in. *BBC News.* Retrieved from http://news.bbc.co.uk/1/hi/magazine/7206663.stm.

Ronksley, P.E., Brien, S.E., Turner, B.J., et al. (2011). Association of alcohol consumption with selected cardiovascular disease outcomes: A systematic review and meta-analysis. *BMJ, 342,* d671.

Ronksley, P.E., Brien, S.E., Turner, B.J., et al. (2012, 21 March). Using imperfect scientific evidence: nuance or rejection? *BMJ,* Rapid Response. Retrieved from http://www.bmj.com/content/342/bmj.d671?tab=responses.

Room, R. (1984). Alcohol control and the field of public health. *Annual Review of Public Health, 5,* 293–317.

Room, R. (1991). Social science research and alcohol policy making. In P. Roman (ed.), *Alcohol: The Development of Sociological Perspectives on Use and Abuse* (pp. 315–39). New Brunswick, NJ: Rutgers Center of Alcohol Studies.

Room, R. (1996). Alcohol consumption and social harm: Conceptual issues and historical perspectives. *Contemporary Drug Problems, 23,* 373–88.

Room, R. (2000). Concepts and items in measuring social harm from drinking. *Journal of Substance Abuse, 12,* 93–111.

Room, R., Babor, T., and Rehm, J. (2005). Alcohol and public health. *The Lancet,* 365, 519–30.

Room, R., Jernigan, D., Carlini-Marlatt, B., et al. (2002). *Alcohol in Developing Societies: A Public Health Approach.* Helsinki, Finland: Finnish Foundation for Alcohol Studies.

Rorabaugh, W.J. (2003). Consumption of alcohol per capita, United States. In J.S. Blocker, D.M. Fahey, and I.R. Tyrrell (eds), *Alcohol and Temperance in Modern History: A Global Encyclopedia* (pp. 23–4). Santa Barbara, CA: ABC-CLIO.

Rosenthal, J., Christianson, A., and Cordero, J. (2005). Fetal alcohol syndrome prevention in South Africa and other low-resource countries. *American Journal of Public Health, 95*(7), 1099–101.

Rosenthal, M.P. (1988). The minimum drinking age for young people: An observation. *The Dickinson Law Review, 92,* 649–63.

Rossow, I., Romelsjö, A., and Leifman, H. (1999). Alcohol abuse and suicidal behaviour in young and middle aged men: Differentiating between attempted and completed suicide. *Addiction, 94*(8), 1199–207.

The Royal Borough of Windsor and Maidenhead (2012). Trading standards—Frequently asked questions. Retrieved from http://www.rbwm.gov.uk/web/ts_trading_stds_faq_27879.htm.

Royal College of Physicians. (1987). *The Medical Consequences of Alcohol Abuse: A Great and Growing Evil.* London: Author.

Royal College of Physicians. (2011). The evidence base for alcohol guidelines. Evidence submitted to the UK Parliament. Retrieved from http://www.publications.parliament.uk/pa/cm201012/cmselect/cmsctech/writev/1536/ag22.htm.

Rush, B. (1785). *An Inquiry into the Effects of Ardent Spirits upon the Human Body and Mind: With an Account of The Means of Preventing, and of the Remedies for Curing Them.* Reprint. Exeter, NH: Richardson.

Saltz, R.F. (2007). How do college students view alcohol prevention policies? *Journal of Substance Use*, *12*(6), 419–26.

Saltz, R.F., and Fell, J.C. (2012). Balancing cost and benefits of the Minimum Legal Drinking Age: A response to Cook and Gearing. In H.R. White and D.L. Rabiner (eds), *College Drinking and Drug Use* (pp. 294–300). New York: The Guilford Press.

Samarasinghe, D. (2006). Sri Lanka: Alcohol now and then. *Addiction*, *101*, 626–8.

Sampson, P.D., Streissguth, A.P., Bookstein, F.L., et al. (1997). Incidence of fetal alcohol syndrome and prevalence of alcohol-related neurodevelopmental disorder. *Teratology*, *56*(5), 317–26.

Sanders, J.L. (2011). Commentary: What might have been: Sullivan may have impacted modern prenatal alcohol research under different circumstances. *International Journal of Epidemiology*, *40*(2), 283–5.

Sandy, A. (2011, 11 August). Glass ban fails to prevent 50 glassings at nightclubs across Queensland. *The Courier-Mail*. Retrieved from http://www.couriermail.com.au/news/queensland/glass-ban-fails-to-prevent-50-glassings-at-nightclubs-across-queensland/story-e6freoof-1226112677889.

Sapru, R.K. (2010). *Public Policy: Art and Craft of Policy Analysis.* New Delhi: PHI Learning.

Sayal, K. (2007). Alcohol consumption in pregnancy as a risk factor for later mental health problems. *Evidence Based Mental Health*, *10*, 98–100.

Schooner set to join pint after drinks measures review. (2011, 4 January). *BBC News*. Retrieved from http://www.bbc.co.uk/news/uk-12113880.

Schooners to be served. (2011, 18 August). *Metro*. Retrieved from http://www.metro.co.uk/news/872704-schooners-to-be-served-in-british-pubs-heineken-and-amstel-lead-way.

Schrad, M.L. (2010). *The Political Power of Bad Ideas: Networks, Institutions, and the Global Prohibition Wave.* Oxford, UK: Oxford University Press.

Schroedel, J.R., and Fiber, P. (2001). Punitive versus public health oriented responses to drug use by pregnant women. *Yale Journal of Health Policy, Law, and Ethics*, *1*, 217–35.

Schuckit, M.A., Smith, T.L., and Landi, N.A. (2000). The 5-year clinical course of high-functioning men with DSM-IV alcohol abuse or dependence. *The American Journal of Psychiatry*, *157*(12), 2028–35.

Schulte, G. (2012, 30 April). Beer companies seek dismissal of reservation suit. *Associated Press*. Retrieved from http://www.google.com/hostednews/ap/article/ALeqM5hyhRhaNpwGH_28yqUFmJFhTdXO9A?docId=331c2ae0f60 14a719d218382e2a6ec99.

Scott, J.C. (1990). *Domination and the Arts of Resistance: Hidden Transcripts*. New Haven, CT: Yale University Press.

The Scottish Government (2012). Alcohol: Research and publications. Retrieved from http://www.scotland.gov.uk/topics/Health/health/Alcohol/resources.

Seitz, H.K., and Becker, P. (2007). Alcohol metabolism and cancer risk. *Alcohol Research and Health*, *30*(1), 38–47.

Selvanathan, S., and Selvanathan, E.A. (2005). *The Demand for Alcohol, Tobacco and Marijuana: International Evidence*. Aldershot, UK: Ashgate.

Seneviratne, K. (2008, 23 January). Sri Lanka's Buddhist monks fight against tobacco and alcohol abuse. *Noticias Financieras*, p. 1. Retrieved from www.proquest.com.

Severson, K. (2011, 28 September). States putting hopes in "bottoms up" to help the bottom line. *New York Times*, p. A1. Retrieved from http://www.nytimes.com/2011/09/29/us/alcohol-laws-eased-to-raise-tax-money.html?pagewanted=all.

Shaffer, H.J., Nelson, S.E., LaPlante, D.A., et al. (2007). The epidemiology of psychiatric disorders among repeat DUI offenders accepting a treatment-sentencing option. *Journal of Consulting and Clinical Psychology*, *75*(5), 795–804.

Sharma, M. (2004). Organizing community action for prevention and control of alcohol and drug abuse. *Journal of Alcohol and Drug Education*, *48*(2), 1–4.

Sharma, M., and Branscum, P. (2010). Editorial: Is Alcoholics Anonymous effective? *Journal of Alcohol and Drug Education*, *54*(3), 3–6.

Shaw, D. (2012, 31 May). David Nutt suggests alcohol sensors "in every car." *BBC News*. Retrieved from http://www.bbc.co.uk/news/uk-18270234.

Shropshire Community Health NHS Trust (2011). Tips for cutting down on your drinking. Retrieved from http://www.healthytelford.nhs.uk/rte.asp?id=116.

Shults, R.A., Elder, R.W., Sleet, D.A., et al. (2001). Reviews of evidence regarding interventions to reduce alcohol-impaired driving. *American Journal of Preventive Medicine*, *21*(4S), 66–88.

Sidlow, E., and Henschen, B. (2009). *America at Odds* (6th ed.). Bellmont, CA: Wadsworth, Cengage Learning.

Single, E., Robson, L., Rehm, J., and Xie, X. (1999). Morbidity and mortality attributable to alcohol, tobacco, and illicit drug use in Canada. *American Journal of Public Health*, *89*(3), 385–90.

Smart, R.G., Adlaf, E.M., and Walsh, G.W. (1994). The relationships between declines in drinking and alcohol problems among Ontario students: 1979–1991. *Journal of Studies on Alcohol, 55*, 338–41.

Smith, R., and Christian, D. (1984). *Bread and Salt: A Social and Economic History of Food and Drink in Russia.* Cambridge, UK: Cambridge University Press.

Smith, D.W. (1979). The fetal alcohol syndrome. *Hospital Practice, 14*(10), 121–8.

Smith, G.S., Branas, C.C., and Miller, T.R. (1999). Fatal nontraffic injuries involving alcohol: A meta-analysis. *Annals of Emergency Medicine, 33*, 659–68.

Smith, R.A., Hingson, R.W., Morelock, S., et al. (1984). Legislation raising the legal drinking age in Massachusetts from 18 to 20: Effect on 16 and 17 year-olds. *Journal of Studies on Alcohol, 45*(6), 534–9.

Smith-Warner, S.A., Spiegelman, D., Yaun, S.S., et al. (1998). Alcohol and breast cancer in women: A pooled analysis of cohort studies. *Journal of the American Medical Association, 279*(7), 535–40.

Smithers, R. (2011, 4 January). Pubs allowed to serve alcohol in smaller glasses. *The Guardian.* Retrieved from http://www.guardian.co.uk/society/2011/jan/04/pubs-serve-alcohol-smaller-glasses?INTCMP=ILCNETTXT3487.

Smithers, R. (2009, 26 March). Britain near top of Europe's teen binge-drinking league. *The Guardian.* Retrieved from http://www.guardian.co.uk/uk/2009/mar/26/teenage-drinking-survey.

Smyth, A. (2004). Introduction. In A. Smyth (ed.), *A Pleasing Sinne: Drink and Conviviality in Seventeenth Century England.* Cambridge, UK: D.S. Brewer.

Snow, D.L., Sullivan, T.P., Swan, S.C., et al. (2006). The role of coping and problem drinking in men's abuse of female partners: Test of a path model. *Violence and Victims, 21*(3), 267–85.

Sood, B., Delaney-Black, V., Covington, C., et al. (2001). Prenatal alcohol exposure and childhood behavior at age 6 to 7 years: I. Dose-response effect. *Pediatrics, 108*(2), e34.

South Dakota v. Dole 483 US 203; 107 S.Ct. 2793; 97 L.Ed. 2d 171 (1987).

Sridhar, D. (2012). Regulate alcohol for global health. *Nature, 482*, 302.

Stade, B., Ali, A., Bennett, D., et al. (2009). The burden of prenatal exposure to alcohol: Revised measurement of cost. *The Canadian Journal of Clinical Pharmacology, 16*, e91–e102.

Staines, G.L., Magura, S., Foote, J., et al. (2001). Polysubstance use among alcoholics. *Journal of Addictive Diseases, 20*(4), 53–69.

Statham, D.J., Connor, J.P., Kavanagh, D.J., et al. (2011). Measuring alcohol craving: Development of the Alcohol Craving Experience questionnaire. *Addiction, 106*(7), 1230–38.

Staudenmeier, W.J. (2011). Alcohol-related windows on Simmel's social world. In P. Kivisto (ed.), *Social Life: Classical and Contemporary Theory Revisited* (5th ed.) (pp. 113–40). Thousand Oaks, CA: Pine Forge Press.

Stephens, O.H., and Scheb, J.M. (2012). *American Constitutional Law: Sources of Power and Restraint* (5th ed.). Boston, MA: Wadsworth Cengage Learning.

Stevens, A. (2007). Survival of the ideas that fit: An evolutionary analogy for the use of evidence in policy. *Social Policy and Society*, *6*(1), 25–35.

Stevenson, J.S. (2005). Alcohol use, misuse, abuse, and dependence in later adulthood. *Annual Review of Nursing Research*, *23*, 245–80.

Stevenson, J.S., and Masters, J.A. (2005). Predictors of alcohol misuse and abuse in older women. *Journal of Nursing Scholarship*, *37*(4), 329–35.

Stockley, C., and Saunders, J.B. (2010). The biology of intoxication. In A. Fox and M. MacAvoy (eds), *Expressions of Drunkenness: Four Hundred Rabbits* (pp. 13–52). New York: Routledge.

Stockwell, R., Greer, A., Fillmore, K., et al. (2012, 21 January). Moderate alcohol consumption and health benefits: How good is the science? *BMJ*, Rapid Response. Retrieved from http://www.bmj.com/content/342/bmj.d671?tab=responses.

Stockwell T., and Grunewald, P. (2004). Controls on the physical availability of alcohol. In N. Heather and T. Stockwell (eds), *The Essential Handbook of Treatment and Prevention of Alcohol Problems* (pp. 213–34). Chichester, UK: John Wiley and Sons.

Stokkeland, K., Brandt, L., Ekbom, A., et al. (2006). Morbidity and mortality in liver diseases in Sweden 1969–2001 in relation to alcohol consumption. *Scandinavian Journal of Gastroenterology*, *41*, 463–8.

STOP Underage Drinking Act passes House. (2006, 14 November). *The Chattanoogan*. Retrieved from http://www.chattanoogan.com/2006/11/14/96713/STOP-Underage-Drinking-Act-Passes.aspx.

Streissguth, A.P., Bookstein, F.L., Barr, H.M., et al. (2004). Risk factors for adverse life outcomes in fetal alcohol syndrome and fetal alcohol effects. *Journal of Developmental and Behavioral Pediatrics*, *25*, 228–38.

Sullivan, W.C. (1899). A note on the influence of maternal inebriety on the offspring. *Journal of Mental Science*, *45*, 489–503.

Surgeon on glass bottle "weapon." (2003, 24 October). *BBC News*. Retrieved from http://news.bbc.co.uk/1/hi/wales/3211769.stm.

Svensson, J. (2012). Alcohol consumption and harm among adolescents in Sweden: Is smuggled alcohol more harmful? *Journal of Child and Adolescent Substance Abuse*, *21*(2), 167–80.

Swedish alcohol intake hikes after EU entry. (2012, 28 April). *The Local*. Retrieved from http://www.thelocal.se/40524/20120428.

Sweden: Bratt Resigns. (1928, 27 August). *Time*. Retrieved from http://www.time.com/time/magazine/article/0,9171,928887,00.html.

Sweden may cut alcohol tax. (2004, 7 May). *Nordic Business Report*, p. 1. Retrieved from www.proquest.com.

Szabo, G. (1997). Alcohol's contribution to compromised immunity. *Alcohol Health and Research World*, *21*, 30–41.

Szalavitz, M. (2012a, 3 May). DSM-5 debate: Committee backs off some changes, reopens comments. *Time: Healthland*. Retrieved from http://healthland.time.

com/2012/05/03/dsm-5-debate-committee-backs-off-some-changes-re-opens-comments.

Szalavitz, M. (2012b, 14 May). DSM-5 could mean 40% of college students are alcoholics. *Time*. Retrieved from http://healthland.time.com/2012/05/14/dsm-5-could-mean-40-of-college-students-are-alcoholics/?iid=hl-main-mostpop1.

Tait, C.J. (2008). Simmering outrage during an "epidemic" of fetal alcohol syndrome. *Canadian Woman Studies*, *26*(3/4), 69–76.

Temkin, D., and Roellke. C. (2009). Federal educational control in No Child Left Behind: Implications of two court challenges. In J.K. Rice and C. Roellke (eds), *High Stakes Accountability: Implications for Resources and Capacity* (pp. 225–50). Charlotte, NC: information Age Publishing.

Temperance and compassion. (2010, 3 October). *The Sunday Times*. Retrieved from http://sundaytimes.lk/101003/Editorial.html.

Temperance in Sweden. (1853, 26 October). *Western Luminary*, *8*(17), p. 3. Retrieved from www.proquest.com.

Testa, M., Fillmore, M.T., Norris, J., et al. (2006). Understanding alcohol expectancy effects: Revisiting the placebo condition. *Alcoholism: Clinical and Experimental Research*, *30*(2), 339–48.

Testa, M., Quigley, B.M., and Leonard, K.E. (2003). Does alcohol make a difference? Within-participants comparison of incidents of partner violence. *Journal of Interpersonal Violence*, *18*, 735–43.

Thadeusz, F. (2009, 24 December). Alcohol's Neolithic origins: Brewing up a civilization. *Der Spiegel*. Retrieved from http://www.spiegel.de/International/zeitgeist/0,1518,668642,00.html.

Thaler, R.H., and Sunstein, C.R. (2008). *Nudge: Improving Decisions about Health, Wealth, and Happiness*. New Haven, CT: Yale University Press.

Thamarangsi, T. (2008). *Alcohol Policy Process in Thailand*. PhD Thesis, Massey University, Auckland, New Zealand.

Thavorncharoensap, M., Teerawattananon, Y., Yothasamut, J., et al. (2010). The economic costs of alcohol consumption in Thailand, 2006. *BMC Public Health*, *10*(323), 1–12.

The hemisphere: End of the anti-saloon act. (1959). *Time*, *74*(24), 14 December.

Thom, B. (2007). Alcohol: Protecting the young, protecting society. In B. Thom, R. Sales, and J.J. Pearce (eds), *Growing Up with Risk* (pp. 241–58). Bristol, UK: The Policy Press.

Thompson, D. (2012a, 17 May). Four out of ten students could be turned into "alcoholics" next year. Is that fair? *The Telegraph*. Retrieved from http://blogs.telegraph.co.uk/news/damianthompson/100158612/four-out-of-ten-students-could-be-turned-into-alcoholics-next-year-is-that-fair.

Thompson, D. (2012b, 28 May). Addiction: The coming epidemic. *The Telegraph*. Retrieved from http://blogs.telegraph.co.uk/news/damianthompson/100161028/addiction-the-coming-epidemic.

Thompson, P. (1999). *Rum Punch and Revolution: Taverngoing and Public Life in Eighteenth-Century Philadelphia*. Philadelphia, PA: University of Pennsylvania Press.

Thun, M.J., Peto, R., Lopez, A.D., et al. (1997). Alcohol consumption and mortality among middle-aged and elderly US adults. *New England Journal of Medicine, 337*(24), 1705–14.

Tigerstedt, C. (1990). The European Community and the alcohol policy dimension. *Contemporary Drug Problems, 17*, 461–79.

Tigerstedt, C. (1999). Alcohol policy, public health and Kettil Bruun. *Contemporary Drug Problems, 26*(2), 209–35.

Toomey, T.L., and Rosenfeld, C. (1996). The minimum legal drinking age. *Alcohol Health and Research World, 20*(4), 213–18.

Toomey, T.L., Nelson, T.F., and Lenk, K.M. (2009). The age-21 minimum legal drinking age: A case study linking past and current debates. *Addiction, 104*, 1958–65.

Tough, S., Clarke, M., and Cook, J. (2007). Fetal Alcohol Spectrum Disorder prevention approaches among Canadian physicians by proportion of Native/ Aboriginal patients: Practices during the preconception and prenatal periods. *Journal of Maternal and Child Health, 11*, 385–93.

Transchel, K. (2003). Alcohol and temperance in the Soviet Union and Russia since 1917. In J.S. Blocker, D.M. Fahey, and I.R. Tyrrell (eds), *Alcohol and Temperance in Modern History: A Global Encyclopedia* (pp. 579–82). Santa Barbara, CA: ABC-CLIO.

Transchel, K. (2006). *Under the Influence: Working-class Drinking, Temperance, and Cultural Revolution in Russia, 1895–1932*. Pittsburgh, PA: The University of Pittsburgh Press.

Treml, V.G. (1997). Soviet and Russian statistics on alcohol consumption and abuse. In J.L. Bobadilla, C.A. Costello, and F. Mitchell (eds), *Premature Death in the New Independent States* (pp. 220–38). Washington, D.C.: National Academy Press.

Treuthart, M.P. (2005). Lowering the bar: Underage drinking. *Journal of Legislation and Public Policy, 9*(1), 101–73.

Tsai, J., Floyd, R.L., Green, P.P., and Boyle, C.A. (2007). Patterns and average volume of alcohol use among women of childbearing age. *Journal of Maternal and Child Health, 11*, 437–45.

Tyrrell, I.R. (1991). *Woman's World/Woman's Empire: The Woman's Christian Temperance Union in International Perspective, 1880–1930*. Chapel Hill, NC: The University of North Carolina Press.

United Nations Office on Drugs and Crime (2009). *Guide to Implementing Family Skills Training Programmes for Drug Abuse Prevention*. Vienna, Austria: Author. Retrieved from http://www.unodc.org/pdf/youthnet/family%20based/ FINAL_ENGLISH_version%20for%20PRINTING%20received%20120209. pdf.

Uradnik, K. (2011). Drinking age. In K. Uradnik, L.A. Johnson, and S. Hower (eds), *Battleground: Government and Politics* (vol. 1) (pp. 170–74). Santa Barbara, CA: ABC-CLIO.

Urbina, I. (2012, 11 May). Addiction diagnoses may rise under guideline changes. *New York Times*, p. A11. Retrieved from http://www.nytimes.com/2012/05/12/us/dsm-revisions-may-sharply-increase-addiction-diagnoses.html?pagewanted=1&_r=1.

US Department of Health and Human Services (2008). *Alcohol: A Women's Health Issue*. Washington, DC: Author, National Institutes of Health, and National Institute on Alcohol Abuse and Alcoholism. Retrieved from http://pubs.niaaa.nih.gov/publications/brochurewomen/women.htm.

US Department of Justice (2000). *Sourcebook of Criminal Justice Statistics*. Washington, DC: US Department of Justice, Bureau of Justice Statistics.

US General Accounting Office (1987). *Drinking-Age-Laws: An Evaluation Synthesis of their Impact on Highway Safety*. Washington, DC: Author.

US Surgeon General releases advisory on alcohol use in pregnancy. (2005, 21 February). Washington, DC: US Department of Health and Human Services. Retrieved from http://www.surgeongeneral.gov/news/2005/02/sg02222005.html.

Vågerö, D. (2011). Alexandr Nemtsov's pioneering work on alcohol in modern Soviet and Russian History. In A. Nemtsov, *A Contemporary History of Alcohol in Russia* (pp. 13–32) (H.M. Goldfinger and A. Stickley, trans.). Stockholm. Sweden: Sodertorns hogskola.

Varvasovszky, Z., and McKee, M. (1998). An analysis of alcohol policy in Hungary. Who's in charge? *Addiction*, *93*(12), 1815–27.

Voas, R.B., and Fell, J.C. (2010). Preventing alcohol-related problems through health policy research. *Alcohol Research and Health*, *33*, 18–28.

Voas, R.B., Tippetts, A.S., and Fell, J.C. (2003). Assessing the effectiveness of minimum legal drinking age and zero tolerance laws in the United States. *Accident Analysis and Prevention*, *35*, 579–87.

Wagenaar, A.C. (1983a). *Alcohol, Young Drivers, and Traffic Accidents*. Lexington, MA: Lexington Books.

Wagenaar, A.C. (1983b). Raising the legal drinking age in Maine: Impact on traffic accidents among young drivers. *International Journal of the Addictions*, *18*(3), 365–77.

Wagenaar, A.C. (1986). Preventing highway crashes by raising the legal minimum age for drinking: The Michigan experience 6 years later. *Journal of Safety Research*, *17*, 101–9.

Wagenaar, A.C. (1993). Research affects public policy: The case of the legal drinking age in the United States. *Addiction*, *88*(s1), 75s–81s.

Wagenaar, A.C., Salois, M.J., and Komro, K.A. (2009). Effects of beverage alcohol price and tax levels on drinking: a meta-analysis of 1003 estimates from 112 studies. *Addiction*, *104*, 179–90.

Wagenaar, A.C., and Toomey, T.L. (2002). Effects of minimum drinking age laws: Review and analyses of the literature from 1960 to 2000. *Journal of Studies on Alcohol, s14*, 206–25.

Wainwright, M. (2012, 22 March). Alcohol abuse contributes to big rise in deaths from liver disease. *The Guardian*. Retrieved from http://www.guardian.co.uk/society/2012/mar/22/alcohol-rise-deaths-liver-disease.

Walker, J.L. (1969). The diffusion of innovations among the American states. *The American Political Science Review, 63*(3), 880–99.

Walker, R. (1989). *The 7 Points of Alcoholics Anonymous*. Center City, MN: Hazelden Publishing.

Wallack, L. (2007). A community approach to the prevention of alcohol-related problems: The San Francisco experience. *International Quarterly of Community Health Education, 26*(2), 109–26.

Wanberg, K.W., Timken, D.S., and Milkman, H.B. (2010). *Driving with Care: Education and Treatment of the Underage Impaired Driving Offender*. Thousand Oaks, CA: SAGE.

Warner, J. (1994a). Resolv'd to drink no more: Addiction as a preindustrial construct. *Journal of Studies on Alcohol and Drugs*, 55, 685–91.

Warner, J. (1994b). In another city, in another time: Rhetoric and the creation of a drug scare in eighteenth-century London. *Contemporary Drug Problems, 21*(Fall), 485–511.

Warner, J. (1998). Historical perspectives on the shifting boundaries around youth and alcohol. The example of pre-industrial England, 1350–1750. *Addiction, 93*(5), 641–57.

Warren, K.R., and Bast, R.J. (1988). Alcohol-related birth defects: An update. *Public Health Reports, 103*(6), 638–42.

Warren, K.R., and Hewitt, B.G. (2009). Fetal alcohol spectrum disorders: When science, medicine, public policy, and laws collide. *Developmental Disabilities Research Reviews, 15*, 170–75.

Warner, J. (2002). *Craze: Gin and Debauchery in an Age of Reason*. New York: Four Walls Eight Windows.

Weiss, C.H. (1982). Policy research in the context of diffuse decision making. *Journal of Higher Education, 53*(6), 619–39.

Weiss, C.H. (1983). Ideology, interests and information: The basis of policy positions. In D. Callahan and B. Jennings (eds), *Ethics, Social Sciences and Policy Analysis* (pp. 213–45). New York: Plenum Press.

Weiss, C.H. (1999). The interface between evaluation and public policy. *Evaluation*. 5(4), 468–86.

Welch, S., and Thompson, K. (1980). The impact of federal incentives on state policy innovation. *American Journal of Political Science, 24*, 715–29.

White, H.R., and Gorman, D.M. (2000). Dynamics of the drug-crime relationship. In G. LaFree (ed.), *Criminal Justice 2000: The Nature of Crime, Continuity and Change*. Washington, DC: US Department of Justice.

White, H.R., Lee, C., Mun, E.-Y., and Loeber, R. (2012). Developmental patterns of alcohol use in relation to the persistence and desistance of serious violent offending among African American and Caucasian young men. *Criminology*, *50*(2), 391–426.

Widom, C.S., and Hiller-Strumhöfel, S. (2001). Alcohol abuse as a risk factor for and consequence of child abuse. *Alcohol Research and Health*, *25*(1), 52–7.

Williams, A.F., Zador, P.L., Harris, S.S., and Karpf, R.S. (1983). The effect of raising the legal minimum drinking age on involvement in fatal crashes. *Journal of Legal Studies*, *12*, 169–79.

Williams, E.M. (2011). Drinking age. In E.M. Williams and S.J. Carter (eds), *The A-Z Encyclopedia of Food Controversies and the Law* (pp. 118–19). Santa Barbara, CA: ABC-CLIO.

Williams, T. (2012, 5 March). At tribe's door, a hub of beer and heartache. *New York Times*. Retrieved from http://www.nytimes.com/2012/03/06/us/next-to-tribe-with-alcohol-ban-a-hub-of-beer.html?_r=1&pagewanted=all.

Winlow, S., and Hall, S. (2006). *Violent Night: Urban Leisure and Contemporary Culture*. Oxford, UK: Berg Publishers.

Wintour, P. (2010, 9 September). David Cameron's "nudge unit" aims to improve economic behaviour. *The Guardian*. Retrieved from http://www.guardian.co.uk/society/2010/sep/09/cameron-nudge-unit-economic-behaviour.

Wirthman, L. (2012, 27 May). Pine Ridge Indian Reservation is drowning in beer. *Denver Post*. Retrieved from http://www.denverpost.com/opinion/ci_20704990/drowning-beer.

Wolfson, M., and Hourigan, M. (1997). Unintended consequences and professional ethics: Criminalization of alcohol and tobacco use by youth and young adults. *Addiction*, *92*(9), 1159–64.

World Health Organization (2004a). *Global Status Report on Alcohol 2004*. Geneva, Switzerland: Author.

World Health Organization (2004b). *International Statistical Classification of Diseases and Related Health Problems* (10th ed., text rev.). Geneva, Switzerland: Author.

World Health Organization (2007). *Evidence-based Strategies and Interventions to Reduce Alcohol-related Harm: Report by the Secretariat*. Sixtieth World Health Assembly, Provisional Agenda Item 12.7. Retrieved from http://apps.who.int/gb/ebwha/pdf_files/WHA60/A60_14-en.pdf.

World Health Organization (2010). *Global Strategy to Reduce the Harmful Use of Alcohol*. Geneva, Switzerland: Author.

World Health Organization (2011a). Alcohol: Fact sheet. Retrieved from http://www.who.int/mediacentre/factsheets/fs349/en/index.html.

World Health Organization (2011b). *Global Status Report on Alcohol and Health*. Geneva, Switzerland: Author. Retrieved from http://www.who.int/substance_abuse/publications/global_alcohol_report/msbgsruprofiles.pdf.

World Health Organization (2012a). Countries: Haiti. Retrieved from http://www.who.int/countries/hti/en.

World Health Organization (2012b). Countries: Iraq. Retrieved from http://www. who.int/countries/irq/en.

World Health Organization (2012c). Social determinants of health. Retrieved from http://www.who.int/social_determinants/en.

World Health Organization Brief Intervention Study Group (1996). A cross-national trial of brief interventions with heavy drinkers. *American Journal of Public Health*, *86*(7), 948–55.

World Health Organization Regional Office for Europe (2009). *Handbook for Action to Reduce Alcohol-related Harm*. Copenhagen, Denmark: Author.

Xu, X., and Chaloupka, F.J. (2011). The effects of prices on alcohol use and its consequences. *Alcohol Research and Health*, *34*(2), 236–45.

Yanovitzky, I., and Bennett, C. (1999). Media attention, institutional response, and health behavior change: The case of drunk driving, 1978–1996. *Communication Research*, *26*(4), 429–53.

Ye, Y., and Cherpitel, C.J. (2009). Risk of injury associated with alcohol and alcohol-related injury. In C.J. Cherpitel, G. Borges, N. Giesbrecht, et al. (eds), *Alcohol and Injuries: Emergency Department Studies in an International Perspective* (pp. 3–13). Geneva, Switzerland: World Health Organization.

Yeomans, H. (2009). Revisiting a moral panic: Ascetic Protestantism, attitudes to alcohol and the implementation of the Licensing Act 2003. *Sociological Research Online*, *14*(2), 6.

Young, D.J., and Bielinska-Kwapisz, A. (2006). Alcohol prices, consumption, and traffic fatalities. *Southern Economic Journal*, *72*(3), 690–703.

Youngerman, B. (2005). *The Truth about Alcohol*. New York: Facts on File.

"Youth tell their story": Case histories from Maryland report. (1938, 6 June). *Life*, *4*(23), 11–21.

Yu, J., Varone, R., and Shacket, R.W. (1997). *A Fifteen-year Review of Drinking Age Laws: Preliminary Findings of the 1996 New York State Youth Alcohol Survey*. New York: Office of Alcoholism and Substance Abuse.

Yudell, M. (2012, 8 May). Can a Bud boycott help the Pine Ridge Reservation? *Philly.com/Health*. Retrieved from http://www.philly.com/philly/blogs/public_health/150544095.html.

Zimring, F.E., and Hawkins, G. (1992). *The Search for Rational Drug Control*. Cambridge, UK: Cambridge University Press.

Index

abstinence from alcohol 38, 49, 64, 67
  see also temperance
abuse of alcohol 4, 8–9, 15–20
  definition of 8–9
acetaldehyde 16
"addiction" to alcohol 4, 9, 21
agenda-setting 27, 29–30, 36, 89
alcohol
  abuse of 4, 8–9, 15–20
  "addiction" to 4, 9, 21
  benefits of alcohol consumption 13, 20
  cancer and 16, 19
  cardiovascular conditions and 20
  costs to societies of alcohol
      consumption 20–21, 45
  cross-national comparisons of
      consumption rates of 15
  deaths due to 2–4, 13, 19–20, 59, 73,
      87–8, 91–2
  dependence on 9, 15
  disease burden related to 3–4, 19
      see also alcohol, cancer and;
          alcohol, cardiovascular
          conditions and; alcohol, liver
          conditions and; alcohol,
          pneumonia and; alcohol,
          tuberculosis and
  domestic violence and 4
  drinking patterns 15–18, 47–52, 76–82
  "expectancies" 50–51
  gender and 14–15, 44, 48, 60, 65, 69,
      72, 80
  genetic factors and 15–16
  guidelines about consumption of
      13–14
  harmful use of 9
  homicides and 4, 59, 109
  industry, alcohol 6, 30–31, 39–40, 53,
      68, 94–5, 105–6
  liver conditions and 19, 73

misuse, alcohol
  definitions of 10, 13–14
  patterns of 15–17
  policies targeting 25–26
mortality related to *see* deaths due to
Native Americans and 5–7, 16, 40,
      47–8
  see also Oglala Sioux Nation
pneumonia and 4, 19
prenatal exposure to 4, 5, 17, 20, 52,
      77
  see also fetal alcohol syndrome
      (FAS)
suicides and 4, 59, 87
taxes on 18, 21–6, 30, 36, 43, 45,
      52–4, 61–2, 73–5, 105
traffic accidents, alcohol-involved 1,
      40, 85–102
trends in consumption of 15, 17–18,
      54, 73
tuberculosis and 4–5, 19
violent victimizations and 1, 4, 45, 48,
      51, 59, 109
Alcohol Measures for Public Health
      Research Alliance (AMPHORA)
      22
Alcohol Policy Network in Europe 52
Alcoholics Anonymous (AA) 25
alcoholism 9, 16, 21
ale 23, 43–6, 48, 82
alehouses 23, 48
  see also bars; inns; pubs; saloons;
      shebeens; taverns
All-Union Voluntary Temperance
      Promotion Society 61
American Medical Association 21
American Prohibition *see* Prohibition Era
      in the US
American Psychiatric Association 9

see also Diagnostic and Statistical
   Manuel of Mental Disorders
American Temperance Foundation 37
Amethyst Initiative 96
apartheid in South Africa 48, 65
archaeological evidence about alcohol
   use 13
Australia 1, 20, 37, 69, 80, 105–6, 108
Austria 18

Band of Hope 37
bars 48–9, 81–2, 99, 109
   see also alehouses; inns; pubs;
      saloons; shebeens; taverns
beer 4–7, 14, 24, 43– 6, 72, 75, 78–82,
   87, 99
Behavioural Insight Team 79
Bermuda 2–3, 16
binge drinking 9, 15, 35, 46–9, 51, 77,
   80–81
   definition of 9, 35
blood-alcohol limit 1, 52
   in Canada 1
   see also zero-tolerance laws
Bolshevik Revolution 58
Bratt, Ivan 72–3, 106
Brazil 1, 108–10
Britain, Great *see* United Kingdom
Bruun, Kettil 21–3
Buddhism 63–8

Cameron, David 1
Campaign for Real Ale (CAMRA) 82
Canada 1, 20, 24, 37, 54, 69, 101
Canada Temperance Act 37
cancer and alcohol consumption 16, 19
Centers for Disease Control and
   Prevention (CDC) 87, 101
China 13, 17, 54
Christianity 23, 63, 65, 68, 104
Congress *see* US Congress
Constitution, US *see* US Constitution
corporate responsibility 6
costs to societies of alcohol consumption
   20–21, 45
crack-cocaine epidemic of the 1980s 46,
   89

Denmark 75
dependence on alcohol 9, 15
depression 17
Diadema, Brazil 108–10
*Diagnostic and Statistical Manual of
   Mental Disorders* 8–9
   fourth edition of (*DSM-IV*) 8–9
   proposals for fifth edition of (*DSM-5*)
      9
diffusion *see* policy diffusion
Directorate-General for Health and
   Consumer Protection (DG
   SANCO) 52, 77–8
doctors *see* physicians
drink driving *see* driving, alcohol-impaired
drinking patterns 15–18, 47–52, 76–82
driving, alcohol-impaired 1, 6–7, 10, 40,
   52, 55, 73, 75, 85–102
drugs, illicit 16–17, 22, 38–9, 46, 89
drunk driving *see* driving, alcohol-
   impaired
Dutch government *see* Netherlands

educational campaigns about alcohol's
   harms 25, 105
Eighteenth Amendment to the US
   Constitution 8, 23–4
   see also Prohibition Era in the US
enforcement of alcohol policies 36, 40, 98,
   101, 109
Estonia 75
European Commission 2, 22, 52, 74, 77–8
European Court of Justice 74, 78
European integration, effects on Swedish
   alcohol policies of 71, 74–8
European Union (EU) 2, 74–6, 87
"evidence-based" programs or policies
   2–3, 27–33, 38–40, 69, 103–7
   see also "what works" literature
excise taxes *see* taxes on alcohol
"expectancies" 50–51

fetal alcohol syndrome (FAS) 5, 20
   economic costs of 20
   see also alcohol, prenatal exposure to
Fielding, Henry 43
Finland 18, 24, 37, 54, 72, 75

First World War *see* World War I
"foreignness" of alcoholic beverages 45,
    63–6
Fourteenth Amendment to the US
    Constitution 95
France 15, 49, 58, 73, 76–7

gender and alcohol 14–15, 44, 48, 60, 65,
    69, 72, 80
"gin craze" 43–6, 66, 104–5
Gin Lane 43–6
Gladwell, Malcolm 49–50
glasnost 61–2, 67
globalization 2, 51–3, 76–8, 83–4, 103–4
Gorbachev, Mikhail 59–63, 69, 105
guidelines for alcohol consumption 13–14

Hammurabi, Ancient Babylonian Code
    of 23
harm reduction approach 22–3
harmful use of alcohol, definition of 9
health benefits of alcohol consumption 20
Heath, Dwight B. 49
Hogarth, William 43–6
Holland *see* Netherlands
homebrewed alcohol *see* moonshine
Hong Kong 2, 18
House of Representatives *see* US House of
    Representatives
    see also US Congress
Hungary 37

illicit drugs 16–17, 22, 38–9, 46, 89
implementation 32, 40, 53, 61–2, 70, 98
    definition of 40
"incrementalism" 31, 53–4, 70, 82
India 54
industry, alcohol 6, 30–31, 39–40, 53, 68,
    94–5, 105–6
infrastructure and alcohol policies 55–6
inns 48
    see also alehouses; bars; pubs;
        saloons; shebeens; taverns
International Monetary Fund (IMF) 34
*International Statistical Classification
    of Diseases and Related Health
    Problems (ICD-10)* 9

internationalization of alcohol issues *see*
    globalization
Ireland 2, 15, 52, 80
Islam 15, 49, 65
Italy 49, 76–7, 86

James, William 13

Kenya 1
Kingdon, John 29–30
    see also agenda-setting; "policy
        entrepreneurs"
Kristof, Nicholas 7

labeling of alcoholic beverages 1, 85
Labour, New 28
Lasswell, Harold D. 27–8
Latin America 40, 55
legislative agenda-setting *see* agenda-
    setting
licensing or licensed premises 23, 25,
    45–6, 97–8
Lightner, Candy 88–9
Lindblom, Charles E. 31, 54, 70, 82
liver conditions and alcohol 19, 73

Malaysia 1
masculinity 60, 69
mead 13
Mexico 47–8
Michigan 93–6, 100–101
minimum drinking age laws 85–102
    in Canada 101
    in Greece 86
    in Italy 86
    in Michigan 85–96, 99–102
    in New Zealand 87–96
    in the UK 86, 101
    in the US 87–93
minimum pricing 1, 24
    see also taxes on alcohol
misuse of alcohol 10, 13–17, 25–6
    definitions of 10, 13–14
    patterns of 15–17
    policies targeting 25–6
monopolies, alcohol retail-related 17,
    24–5, 63–4, 73–8, 83

moonshine 59–60, 62, 108
Mothers Against Drunk Driving (MADD)
    55, 88–9, 96
"muddling through" 32

National Institute on Alcohol Abuse and
    Alcoholism (NIAAA) 20, 22
National Minimum Drinking Age Act of
    1984 90–91
National Transportation Safety Board 88
Native Americans 5–7, 16, 40, 47–8
    see also Oglala Sioux Nation
Netherlands 2, 43
New York State 92
New Zealand 24, 80, 96–102
Nicholas II, Tsar 58, 62
Norway 72, 77
"nudge" theory 78–83, 104

Oglala Sioux Nation 5–8, 83, 104

Pan American Health Organization 110
patterns, drinking 15–18, 47–52, 76–82
physicians 21, 25–6
Pine Ridge Reservation *see* Oglala Sioux
    Nation
pints, tradition of drinking in 78, 81–3
policy diffusion 33–5, 37–8, 52, 88–90,
    101, 103–4
"policy entrepreneurs" 30, 35, 65, 106–7
policy implementation *see* implementation
"policy incrementalism" *see*
    "incrementalism"
policy learning 34, 52, 101–2
"policy orientation" 28
policy transfer *see* policy diffusion
political agenda-setting *see* agenda-setting
polysubstance abuse 16–17
post-traumatic stress disorder (PTSD) 17
prescription drugs 17
Presidential Commission on Drunk
    Driving 89
price of alcohol *see* minimum pricing or
    taxes on alcohol
prohibition
    at Pine Ridge Reservation 5–8, 47
    prohibition movements in general
        37–8

prohibition movements in Sri Lanka
    63–70
prohibition movements in Sweden 72
in Russia or the Soviet Union 58–63,
    68–70, 105, 108
    see also Prohibition Era in the US
Prohibition Era in the US 8, 18, 23–4, 47,
    55, 57, 62, 69, 106, 108
public health perspective 21–2, 26, 55,
    71–4, 77–8
public opinion and alcohol policies 54–5,
    61, 76, 82–3, 100–101, 105–6, 109
pubs 48, 50, 80–82, 99, 101
    see also alehouses; bars; inns; saloons;
        shebeens; taverns

randomized controlled trials 32
Reagan, Ronald 89–90
religion and alcohol 47, 49–50, 63–6, 69
    see also Buddhism; Christianity; Islam
Remove Intoxicated Drivers (RID) 88
research evidence and alcohol policies
    see "evidence-based" programs or
        policies
rounds, tradition of drinking in 78–83, 104
Rush, Benjamin 4, 19, 21–2
Russia 58, 62, 69, 72
    historical drinking patterns in 58
    see also Gorbachev, Mikhail; Nicholas
        II, Tsar; prohibition in Russia or
        the Soviet Union; Soviet Union

Sale of Liquor Act of 1989 97
Sale of Liquor Amendment Act of 1999 97
saloons 50
São Paulo 109
    see also alehouses; bars; inns; pubs;
        shebeens; taverns
schooner 81–2
Scotland 1
    see also United Kingdom
Second World War *see* World War II
shebeens 48, 65
    see also alehouses; bars; inns; pubs;
        saloons; taverns
"sly grogging" 108
social determinants of health perspective
    22–3

social harm, definition of 3, 19
South Africa 48, 65,
South Dakota 5, 90–91, 104
South Dakota v. Dole 90–91
Soviet Union 57–63, 67–70, 76, 83, 105,
    108
    see also glasnost; Russia; Stalin,
        Joseph
spirits 43–5, 58, 72–3, 75, 101
    see also "gin craze"
Sri Lanka 63–70, 94, 104, 106
Stalin, Joseph 58
standard drinks 14
    see also guidelines for alcohol
        consumption
Sunstein, Cass 79, 82
Supreme Court, US *see* US Supreme Court
Sweden 24–5, 58, 68, 71–8, 83–4, 90, 103,
    108
    see also Systembolaget, the
Systembolaget, the 73–8

taverns 48
    see also alehouses; bars; inns; pubs;
        saloons; and shebeens
taxes on alcohol 18, 21–6, 30, 36, 43, 45,
    52–4, 61–2, 73–5, 105
temperance 18, 23–4, 37–8, 45, 47, 55,
    63–9, 72–3, 89, 104, 106
    see also abstinence from alcohol
Thailand 21, 53–4, 70
Thaler, Richard 79–82, 104
"third place" 50
Tippling Act of 1751 45–6
traffic accidents, alcohol-involved *see*
    driving, alcohol-impaired
Twenty-sixth Amendment to the US
    Constitution 87, 93
"two communities" thesis 28, 33, 85–6,
    91, 95

underground drinking *see* moonshine
United Kingdom 1, 13–14, 17–19, 28,
    34–5, 37–8, 43–52, 63–9, 78–83,
    101, 104–6
    see also Scotland

United Nations' Office on Drugs and
    Crime 2
United States 4–9, 17–18, 23–4, 35, 39,
    46–7, 55, 57, 62, 65–6, 69, 85–96,
    99–102, 106–7, 108
    Congress 39, 88–90, 96, 101–2
    Constitution of 8, 23–4, 87, 90, 93, 95
    costs of alcohol consumption in 20
    deaths, alcohol-related, in 13
    guidelines regarding alcohol
        consumption in 14
    historical consumption patterns in 18
    House of Representatives 101–2
    minimum drinking age policies in
        85–96, 99–102
    monopolies, alcohol retail-related, in
        24
    policy diffusion in 34
    Prohibition Era in 8, 18, 23–4, 47, 55,
        57, 62, 69, 106, 108
    research on alcohol in 22
    Supreme Court 90
    taxes on alcohol in 21, 23–4, 36
units of alcohol 14
US Congress 39, 88–90, 96, 101–2
    see also US House of Representatives
US Constitution 8, 23–4, 87, 90, 93, 95
    Eighteenth Amendment to 8, 23–4
    Fourteenth Amendment to 95
    Twenty-first Amendment to 90
    Twenty-sixth Amendment to 87, 93
US House of Representatives 101–2
    see also US Congress
US Supreme Court 90
Utah 49–50, 65–6

Vietnam War 87, 93, 99
vodka 58–9, 62
Volstead Act *see* Prohibition Era in the US

Walker, Jack 34
Weiss, Carol H. 29–31, 67, 79, 106–7
"what works" literature 4, 32, 53, 71
    see also "evidence-based" programs or
        policies
Whiteclay, Nebraska 4–7, 83
wine 13–14, 23–4, 52, 75, 81–2

World Health Organization (WHO) 2, 4,
        21–2, 36, 69, 103
    *see also International Statistical
        Classification of Diseases and
        Related Health Problems (ICD-10)*
World Trade Organization (WTO) 34, 90
World War I 37, 58, 60, 72, 80
World War II 18

Yeltsin, Boris 62

zero-tolerance laws 1, 92